T0208582

LABOR LIKE A
GODDESS

A FEARLESS GUIDE TO PREPARING FOR

THE 7 GATES OF TRANSFORMATION

IN PREGNANCY AND BIRTH

ALEXANDRIA MORAN
&
LAUREN MAHANA

BALBOA.PRESS
A DIVISION OF HAY HOUSE

Balboa Press books may be ordered through booksellers or by contacting:

Balboa Press
A Division of Hay House
1663 Liberty Drive
Bloomington, IN 47403
www.balboapress.com
1 (877) 407-4847

Interior and Cover Art Credit: Gina Fuschetto

Print information available on the last page.

ISBN: 978-1-9822-3586-4 (sc)
ISBN: 978-1-9822-3588-8 (hc)
ISBN: 978-1-9822-3587-1 (e)

Library of Congress Control Number: 2019915252

Balboa Press rev. date: 12/18/2019

Praise for Labor Like A Goddess

"*Labor Like A Goddess* restores the ancient wisdom that has been missing in modern day birth literature! Alexandria and Lauren walk you through the transitional gates in preparation for the next phase of your life, step by step. They have added practical tools and thought-provoking questions that will help you embrace the journey and look forward to your labor and birth. You can do this - your power is already within. Allow this book to wake the courage inside as you walk into motherhood. As an educator, this will now be the pre-reading for all of my birth classes."

— Care M. Messer, Founder of the Birth Education Center (www. BirthEducationCenter.com), Birth Educator, Certified Hypnotherapist, Birth & Postpartum Doula

"I wish I had this book when I was pregnant 30 years ago. During my reading, my own labor experiences came rushing back to me and I found myself wondering how things might have unfolded for me if I had this book as a birthing companion. This book discusses, in-depth, all of the essential emotional and spiritual challenges of labor that are not openly acknowledged and addressed in the medical community, with families, friends, and even our partners. Reading this book is the initial step women can take to create that sense of community so necessary to ease the burden of labor and to transform it into a spiritual awakening.

How women cross the threshold from Maiden-to-Mother, influences how they are able to create a secure attachment with their baby. This book provides an essential map for how we begin our life-long journey in creating loving, aware, and securely attached relationships with our children. I am recommending this book to every pregnant client I have, to every pregnant woman I know, as well as to every woman who is thinking about becoming pregnant, or has already birthed her children and wants to better understand her experience and integrate it into her mothering moving forward. Praise to Alexandria Moran and Lauren Mahana!"

— Jane Ryan M.A., LMFT, Intimate Relationships Therapist, Ryan Couples Therapy (www.ryancouplestherapy.com)

"*Labor Like A Goddess* takes you on a journey unlike any other pregnancy and parent-to-be books out there. It is a quest of closing cycles and creating new life and through that, a new world. The authors, while providing the tools and support necessary, challenge their readers to do the transformative work of becoming mother, of becoming parent. This book is an absolute must read for 1st, 2nd, 3rd time parents — never too late to learn how to conquer fear and create new healthy cycles through the birth of a child and their parents!"

— Emily Moy, Birth & Postpartum Doula

"A tremendously insightful guide with an alternate perspective to childbirth than most reads available today! As an expecting mother, the way this book is broken down as both a resource and an interactive workbook has helped me prepare for the upcoming birth of my first daughter. I would recommend *Labor Like a Goddess* to any mother looking for a spiritual yet pragmatic step-by-step approach to easing fears and common concerns associated with many modern-day birthing practices. This book really highlights the invaluable importance of the doula's place in the birthing process."

— Amanda Victoria, first time mother-to-be, New York City

"This is the book I wish I could have had to prepare me for my own birth experiences. It encourages mothers-to-be to get in tune with their inner strengths, fears, and desires and learn how to empower themselves throughout the awesome journey that is the transition into motherhood. As women prepare for this transition, we're often told what expectations we SHOULD have and we neglect our own intuition. This book provides a straightforward, intuitive guide to put mothers-to-be back in touch with their instincts."

— Erin Knittel, LMHC, Psychotherapist specializing in life transitions

For all those who hear the emotional and spiritual calling to surrender to the transformative power of labor. . . May this book be your beacon of light and grounded sounding board as you journey into your own emotional Underworld to birth your baby and yourself as a mother.

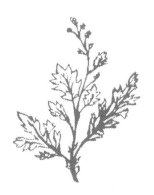

CONTENTS

Introduction

You, the Goddess

So many women have taken the hero's journey, only to find it personally empty . . . women emulated the male heroic journey because there were no other images to emulate.

—*Maureen Murdock*

Woman, you are a Divine birth goddess, and within you is the wisdom and power to manifest the birth experience that your soul has been dreaming into existence. We intend that this book will help you find your inner strength and courage so you may fearlessly walk through the seven physical, emotional, and spiritual Gates of Transformation that await you in labor. Because, the truth is, you are not just birthing your baby . . . You will be birthing your Mother-self too!

Becoming a mother is one of the most significant spiritual rites of passage that most of us will ever experience. The journey of labor and birth offers the incredible opportunity to fully surrender to and merge with our inner Divine self, our own inner goddess—even if for just a brief moment. Our wish for you is that you be fully prepared and educated for not only the physical transformation that awaits in birth, but also the psychological, emotional, and spiritual transformation as well. We hope the wisdom and teachings in this book will illuminate a new way of looking at your labor journey—one that will bring you greater empowerment as you cross the threshold into motherhood.

A Doula's Perspective

This book is written by two professional doulas and modern moms who are deeply concerned about what we see as an alarming trend happening in childbirth. Recent research shows that more than one-third[1] of women feel psychologically and emotionally traumatized by their birth experiences, and many experience some form of postpartum depression or dissatisfaction as a result[2]. These statistics are despite education, birth preparation, and physical readiness. This research mirrors the trends that we see play out anecdotally in our work, and among family and friends. We have noticed that a mother's background, nationality, income level, religion, birth location, birth choices, medical professionals, or the level of support from the immediate family were immaterial in determining her satisfaction with her birth experience. Something deeper was going on in the psyche of a laboring mother, and no one seemed to be talking about it.

As we explored further, we began noticing that all laboring women seemed to face the same seven emotional and spiritual challenges throughout pregnancy and labor:

1. **Fear:** Even the most confident moms find themselves faced with varying degrees of fear throughout pregnancy and birth. The physical fears of body changes, weight gain, the baby's health, possible delivery complications, and lifestyle changes show up in almost all of our clients at some point. Emotional fears of change, motherhood, worthiness, preparedness, overwhelm, the unknown, vulnerability, doubt, loss, and grief also arise—though are often more difficult to detect.

2. **Shame:** Our clients tell us that this the most unexpected experience to show up in the throes of labor, but because shame exists in the womb space, it goes hand-in-hand with birth. Shame around nudity, vulnerability, how labor is experienced, and even unresolved past traumas are often activated with the contracting womb.

3. **Control:** Even the most laidback and relaxed expectant mothers find themselves wrestling with issues of control—of the body, the mind, emotions, and circumstances—because birth requires total surrender to the primal force of nature.

4. **Trust:** Whether it's trusting others, partners, medical attendants, family members, a divine power, or themselves, struggles with trust show up even in the most faithful and hopeful expectant mothers.

When trust issues show up during a vulnerable state such as labor, it can often feel too dangerous or risky to allow trust.

5. **Staying present:** Birth is an intense experience emotionally, physically, and spiritually, so even the most Zen moms-to-be can struggle with staying in the present moment. The temptation to numb or hide can be difficult to avoid.

6. **Perseverance:** When dealing with new and unexpected physical and emotional sensations, it can be difficult to cultivate the fortitude needed to persevere and stay focused on the end goal—a healthy and empowering delivery. Even the most determined moms-to-be can find themselves struggling.

7. **Acceptance:** This challenge is experienced by even the most easygoing moms-to-be, and it often is the root of birth trauma. Acceptance requires an intentional surrender of the basic instinct to survive, which is contrary to both nature and self-preservation.

When these challenges are acknowledged and overcome throughout pregnancy and the labor process, moms describe their births as being "empowering" and "divine" while experiencing a smoother transition into motherhood—even if the medical events that unfolded were traumatic, unexpected, unwanted, or shocking. Even more surprising, we have noticed that many of the women who resisted these seven emotional and spiritual challenges described their births as "traumatic"—even if the medical events unfolded precisely the way they wanted.

Having witnessed and listened to hundreds of birth stories, we realized that labor is so much more than a physical experience—it is an inward transformational journey into the deepest parts of ourselves. As described above, along the way we face seven specific challenges—or as we term them, the seven "Gates of Transformation," and so we developed a mythic story or metaphor and some practical tools to help our moms-to-be navigate the transition from Maiden-to-Mother. As our clients began to understand birth in this way, we noticed how they started to intentionally embrace their own spiritual and emotional transformation and experience labor with more profound satisfaction—no matter what the outcome. Acknowledging and embracing this inner journey is what truly makes an empowered birth.

We would love to share this information with more women, but because we are busy doulas, with a limited amount of births we can support each year, we felt it was important to put these findings into a book, so many more moms-to-be could have access to this transformative and empowering information. Because we are emotional support birth attendants, not doctors or midwives, we leave the medical aspects to the professionals, so we won't be discussing medical specifics throughout this book. Nor will we be discussing stages of labor, physical comfort measures, or laboring positions as these can be found in any number of birth preparation books. Instead, we'll be focusing on what we've found to be missing in the childbirth preparation arena—practical tools for dealing with the emotional and spiritual challenges and sacrifices that show up in pregnancy and labor.

If we aren't afraid to tell it like it is and push a little tough love into the space, it's because we know that this is an entirely different way to look at pregnancy, childbirth, and your own emotional Underworld, so we want to make sure you "get it." When all is said and done, our goal is to encourage you to reach for a deeper level of self-mastery and healing so you can be empowered to release your old Maiden-self to birth your Mother-self into the world! We believe in your power, strength, courage, and ability to have the emotionally and spiritually empowered birth you are longing for.

The Goddess Story

Throughout this book, we'll be sharing the same metaphorical story that we use to help our moms-to-be understand the deeper challenges of childbirth and labor. The myth tells the journey of the Maiden Goddess and how she powerfully transforms herself into Mother by venturing into the unknown Underworld, bravely walking through the seven Gates of Transformation, and making seven specific sacrifices along the way. This tale is loosely based on the ancient Sumerian myth of the Goddess Innana and her journey into the Underworld, where she allows herself to die and must find the inner power to resurrect herself stronger than ever. Like Innana, our Maiden Goddess must also discover her strength, courage, trust, fortitude, and self-mastery on her own metaphorical adventure of the emotional and psychological journey into motherhood—allowing her old self to die away so she can resurrect as Mother Goddess.

As doulas, we've found that the story of the Maiden Goddess offers moms-to-be a powerful blueprint for understanding labor as a spiritual journey to help them recognize the emotional sacrifices that arise and learn the practical tools they need to walk through the Gates of Transformation into motherhood. Each gate is rooted in emotional sacrifice and reward, which we'll be sharing with you in the following chapters:

1. The Gate of Courage and Sovereignty
2. The Gate of Vulnerability
3. The Gate of Expectations
4. The Gate of Embodiment
5. The Gate of Sacred Partnership
6. The Gate of Fortitude
7. The Gate of Intentional Surrender

As each gate appears, the Maiden Goddess discovers she must face her own resistance to the sacrifices being asked of her. She doesn't take anything at face value, but rather questions the Gatekeeper, takes a step back to really understand the purpose of the sacrifice, and then makes her choice to move forward. She teaches us that being mindful, asking questions, and going within for answers is the necessary work to move through our Underworld journey to the Maiden death with empowerment, rather than trauma.

Recognizing birth as an emotional and spiritual sacrifice can help us piece together why inner symbolic death is necessary for growth. The comforts the Maiden Goddess must sacrifice at each gate represent the hindrances that hold her back from shifting into a new experience of life. Each item she gives away is a metaphorical coping tool that has helped her through maidenhood: a sword to feel protected, a cloak to cover her, a map to give her purpose, and so on. As laboring women, we are also asked to surrender our emotional, psychological, and physical coping tools so we can feel prepared to allow our inner Maiden—the lifestyle we lived before having children—to die away at the final Gate of Motherhood.

We'll be sharing parts of the Maiden Goddess story at the beginning of each chapter, but if you would like to read the story in its entirety, you can find it on our website www.laborlikeagoddess.com. This story is the foundational piece for the rest of the book, and we will reference it often, so you may find it helpful to read this story as often as you can to allow its symbols and metaphors to penetrate your psyche. Some moms-to-be even bring the story to their labors and have their birth partners read it to them when they find themselves fighting their own resistance.

Each chapter also contains Integration Practices—such as self-love exercises, journaling prompts, rituals, and meditations—to help you work through each of your own personal sacrifices and walk through each of the gates with empowerment. These practices are extensive, so please don't feel you need to do them all, but rather focus on those that speak to you. However, it may be helpful to note any practices you resist because these are often the ones with the most medicine and are the most helpful in the end.

Inclusivity and Gender Sensitivity

Although not everyone reading this book will identify as female or mother, the emotional and spiritual shift from pre-baby to life with baby happens for everyone—regardless of gender identity or expression. Throughout this book, we use feminine pronouns and archetypes to tell the Maiden-to-Mother story as a way of describing this major life transformation. However, this journey is also relevant to a non-cis-gender experience, and we hope you can find empowerment in these pages no matter what gender you identify with. Parents-to-be of all identities can discover their story within these pages because the archetype of the Triple Moon Goddess (Maiden-Mother-Crone) embodies the spirit and process of transformation for us all. Though the goddess is traditionally a feminine figure, her power is not just for cis-women— anyone that births a baby walks the same journey through the Gates of Transformation.

The Power of Story as Medicine

Storytelling is distinctly human. Stories can powerfully bind strangers together as one humanity and help us live with a collective understanding. As long as language has existed, humans have been telling stories to help shape culture, define values, set social norms, explain events, and pass down wisdom in a way that is easily understood—even by children. This is why we read stories to children as our first touchstones of communication; they create connection and a sense of belonging to the community, and they help us make sense of a world that can sometimes seem senseless.

The great power of storytellers also comes with great responsibility, because stories are compelling and can be used to spread *love* or create *fear*. As doulas, we can't help but notice how many of our cultural birth stories seem to be rooted in chaos, fear, shame, and trauma, with birthing women feeling out of control and medical professionals saving the day. There is nothing wrong with this, except that it only tells one version of birth—a patriarchal one that can be disempowering to the fortitude and inherent power of a modern-day Maiden transitioning into motherhood.

The truth is, birth is a divinely powerful and empowering experience, and we need more stories that tell us this truth. Stories that reveal strength we never knew we had, a fortitude we didn't know existed and an act of courage that is only told in myths can perhaps be the best medicine needed right now. This is why we have decided to retell the ancient Sumerian story of the Goddess Innana's descent into the Underworld in a modern way. The sacrifice of her worldly goods as she descends through different gates into the Underworld and, ultimately, dies to be reborn is the perfect metaphor for the emotional and spiritual experience of birth. This concept of death and rebirth is so firmly rooted to a woman's journey through the Gates of Transformation that we felt as doulas it perfectly explains what has, until now, been too abstract to understand.

We hope that our version of the Innana story offers you an alternative understanding of birth—one that is rooted in the truth, for the modern-day parent. Giving birth is hard work and requires great emotional sacrifice: a willingness to strip away feelings of safety and comfort to venture into the Underworld of our souls, all in the name of becoming a mother. Birth is the human version of a phoenix rising from the ashes—stronger, more empowered, and more conscious than ever.

Consider this book a Divine call to conscious motherhood through the process of prepared and Divine laboring. Just like the Maiden Goddess in our story, you too will be asked to journey into the Underworld. But instead of a mythical place, you will delve into your own subconscious mind and emotions. You'll be asked to witness your pain, your shame, your fears, and anything that keeps you small. You'll be asked to grow and stretch in ways you didn't think possible. You'll be offered the opportunity to release old coping mechanisms and allow old versions of yourself to die away. In return, you will shape yourself into the kind of mother your child needs to thrive and feel deeply loved. It is a journey of sacrifice, reward, and transformation from Maiden-to-Mother.

It might not always be easy, but it'll be worth it. And we promise you this: if you're willing to shed the old version of yourself, you will find a level of courage, strength, perseverance, and empowerment that will inspire you through the next 18-plus years of motherhood. So, whether this is your first birth or your fifth, think of this book as your guide to help you fearlessly prepare for transformation on all levels into motherhood.

Will you heed the call into the Underworld? Are you ready to become a Mother Goddess?

If so, let's begin . . .

CHAPTER I

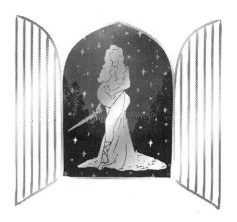

THE JOURNEY FROM MAIDEN TO MOTHER

CROSSING THE GATES OF TRANSFORMATION

Mothers need just as much attention as a newborn because they, too, have just been born.

—*Unknown*

Once upon a time, there was a Maiden Goddess who was young, beautiful, and full of life. She was abundant and happy and lived her days picking flowers, dancing in the sun, making magic with the forest animals, and enjoying amazing sex with her Beloved life partner. She was happy, but couldn't help feeling that something was missing in her life. She felt a deep stirring within—a calling from her womb to create. She longed to become a mother.

One night, she heard the Moon calling to her, telling her that if she wanted to create life, she would need to leave the safety and comfort of her sun-filled world and travel to the depths of the dark Underworld. She would have to sacrifice much, but when she returned, the Moon promised to bless her as a mother.

The Maiden Goddess didn't want to leave her Beloved or the animals or the warmth of the sun. But over the following days, the calling within grew to a roar she could no longer ignore—she longed to become a mother. So, she decided to take the unknown journey into the Underworld.

As she started to pack her bags, she asked herself what necessities she needed to take with her to help keep her safe, protected, and comfortable on the journey ahead. She thought to herself, "Well, of course, I will have to take a sword for protection, my cloak for modesty and warmth, a map so I know where I'm going, and sturdy shoes to help me last the journey." Her bag was packed, and she kissed her Beloved goodbye, knowing she had to make this journey alone.

Birth is a Transformative Journey

Birth is a powerfully transformative experience. As a society, we honor the physical transition with baby showers and registries, birth classes, comfort measures, and push gifts. Birth is a time of pure bliss, but we sometimes neglect the emotional, psychological, and spiritual experiences of transformation that show up throughout pregnancy, labor, and birth, which can be really confusing to a new mom. No one talks about the level of sacrifice and surrender that can stretch the psychological parameters of a laboring mother, nor do we talk about the emotional waves of uncertainty or doubt that most of us experience or how to ride them.

Birth is the most spiritual and paranormal experience we have as humans, aside from death. On the most obvious level, it is literally a spirit merging into the physical, heaven coming to earth. Without the language or understanding to recognize what is happening, this process can bring fear, shame, and resistance. When we are more conscious of what is happening, birth can offer the opportunity for deeply personal, emotional, and spiritual healing for all those present. Shamans and ancient medicine healers understood that labor is one of the most powerful opportunities for a woman to heal and purify herself, her baby, and her lineage, should she choose to embrace it. Each Gate of Transformation that she willingly surrenders to *before* the baby is born releases old patterns forever, so the next generation is free from the burden of battling unhealthy wounds, habits, addictions, or behaviors. A spiritual evolution of sorts is available in every pregnancy and at every labor. However, if we don't realize this opportunity, we may very well miss it or even become traumatized by it.

When we approach birth holistically with preparation, education, support, and understanding, it can be one of the most fulfilling and empowering experiences of our lives. However, when we are unprepared for the transformation, we may fight the sacrifices or even get stuck in psychological trauma. The Maiden Goddess story teaches us that our willingness to surrender to each Gate of Transformation is the key to feeling empowered by our birth experiences and preventing trauma.

When we choose to walk the path of motherhood, we must be willing to let go of the old and allow things to die—even cherished parts of ourselves. Just like the Maiden Goddess, we have to choose to release old ideas, beliefs, thoughts, feelings, and the dynamics of our current Maiden psyche and trust that, in doing so, we will rise like the phoenix from the ashes as something better—the empowered Mother Goddess.

Birth is the Ultimate Act of Feminism

Birth used to be a female-only event where the women of the village would gather together to dance, adorn, massage, entertain, support, and offer love to a laboring woman as she facilitated her baby's spiritual entry into the physical world through labor. As the tribal sisterhood supported the emotional needs of the laboring woman, encouraging her to bravely walk through her own Gates of Transformation, midwives would attend to the medical needs of the mother and baby. It was a collective female effort to birth the new baby *and* a new mother into the village.

As we moved away from tribal living and more into our modern-day, individualized society, we started to lose the female support of this sisterhood. Midwives began to be replaced by male doctors in hospitals, and our birth culture shifted from matriarchal to patriarchal. Suddenly, women were looking to men for answers on how to labor, and because these men did not have generations of wisdom, comfort measures, body positions, herbs, and tools, they applied what they did know—medicine.

While birth became safer, it became less vibrant, less expressive, more controlled, less intuitive, and more procedural. Generation after generation bred the habit of babies being born this way, which started to chip away at our female sense of empowerment, pleasure, purpose, and spiritual journey that birth had always been. Birth suddenly became merely a medical procedure, a means to an end, that focused only on the baby without supporting the woman's own emotional transformation.

Recently, there has been a resurgence in calling on ancient female wisdom about birth with more and more moms advocating traditions like skin-to-skin, delayed cord clamping, home laboring, belly dancing, and doula care (hiring emotionally supportive birth attendants, like us). Yet, we still have a long way to go in re-establishing birth as truly a sacred rite of passage, an act of transformation, and a shift in emotional/spiritual consciousness.

Returning to the essence of birth is a fierce act of feminism for mom, partner, baby, family, medical staff, and society as a whole. This is because, when a woman is supported and empowered in her birth experience, it translates to all other areas of her life, amplifying her ability to consciously and compassionately guide and raise the next generation of humanity.

When we align with our own body's wisdom, trust the good intentions of our medical care providers, walk through each gate willingly, and finally surrender to our own rebirth, we become goddesses in the flesh. And what greater act of feminism is there than that!

When we start to see birth from this perspective, we can cultivate the feminine courage that lives within every mother who has ever been or will ever be. Birth becomes a collective female experience and an energetic and spiritual initiation into the greatest act of sacrifice ever asked of humanity: motherhood.

Gates and Cycles

Because labor and birth is a female journey, it is important to take into consideration the natural cyclical nature of the Divine Feminine. But first, let's define the Divine Feminine: it is the archetypal side of God, Allah, Source, Creation, Divinity, Supreme Being, Higher Power or whatever your call 'All That Is' that is expressed through the feminine qualities of creation, destruction, intuition, connection, sensuality, beauty, nourishment, mothering, compassion, cycles, curves, spirals, and flow. It is the cycle of death and birth most obviously seen through nature. We even call it "Mother Nature" as a way to understand this Divine Feminine energy.

Mother Nature teaches us about the Divine Feminine through her own cycles of the seasons. Each year we witness the metamorphosis of the entire Earth through its own birth-death-rebirth cycle from spring to winter back to spring. Each year a physical, spiritual, and symbolic death occurs as plants die, animals hibernate, and winter freezes all activity; each year rebirth occurs as plants return, animals are born, and harvests are reaped. We learn that nothing ever truly dies but is reborn stronger, healthier as life always returns. The seasons have much to teach us about our own cycles as women and the different stages of life from Maiden-to-Mother-to-Enchantress-to-Crone, mirroring spring to summer to fall to winter.

The Moon, a typically feminine symbol in most of our cultural stories, also has much to teach us about cycles—perhaps more directly than

Earth. Did you know that women bleed for the same number of days that the Moon takes to cycle through all her phases? That is no coincidence. Women are guided by the same Divine Feminine energy as the Moon, and our menstrual cycles often sync with the phases of the Moon. The Dark Moon reflects the bleeding time of menstruation and our desire to just cuddle on the couch and "go dark." The Waxing Moon reflects pre-ovulation and the time to start building energy and desire after a week of bleeding. The Full Moon reflects ovulation when we are at our most fertile and are ready to be seen and adored. The Waning Moon reflects pre-menstruation when we prepare ourselves to go dark again and often feel irritable when we have to be social. The Moon also pulls the tides of the Earth's oceans (water—another feminine symbol) as it pulls the tides of our womb waters. It's no wonder the maternity wards are always busy on a Full Moon, as it conjures a high rise in amniotic water breaking and women going into labor.

When we start to see that we are guided by the same energy that guides the Earth and the Moon, it becomes clear that aligning with that energy makes labor much easier and fighting it can cause problems. It's time to fully embrace the notion that a woman's natural rhythm is to cycle like the Moon, spiral like the tide pools, dance with leaves on the wind, deepen into the mud of the Earth, expand into the Full Moon, and contract into the Dark Moon—all in harmony with nature.

It is clear that women are anything but linear, especially as we move through the phases of pregnancy, labor, and motherhood. So it is important to note, as we walk through the Gates of Transformation in labor, that just because they are laid out linearly to make a good story, that isn't how we typically experience the gates. We might skip gates, return to gates we already went through, spiral through the same gate over and over again, or find ourselves going through multiple gates all at once. That is perfectly natural and a validation that we are in our Divine Feminine rhythm. It may be tempting to approach the gates as we would a shopping list, checking off each item one at a time. However, it is important to allow the Divine Feminine to guide us. The gates, birth, labor, pregnancy, and motherhood all rely on our ability to tap into this natural Mother Earth energy and sacrifice any sense of one-dimensional, linear thinking.

Motherhood: Great Sacrifice and Great Reward

If we haven't made it obvious so far, we hope it is now: the journey to becoming a mother is a sacred initiation of great sacrifice and reward. Caring for a baby in our wombs for 40 weeks kicks off this initiation with many small, physical sacrifices, starting with our comfort. We usually have to stop drinking alcohol and eating some of our favorite foods. We surrender to sleepless nights, an expanding body, swollen limbs, and physical discomfort. Many times our sacrifices reshape our finances, relationships, and careers, too.

However sacrifice shows up in pregnancy, our world starts to look very different than it once did. That is because the honor of carrying a baby in the womb requires great sacrifice for the baby to be born healthy—a fabulous reward. So, with great sacrifice comes great reward. The same goes for labor, too.

Labor is the next level in this sacred initiation into motherhood. It too asks for great physical sacrifice as the body will have to expand, stretch, and open in ways it has never done before. Most childbirth preparation classes focus on the physical sacrifice by preparing us for labor with education on choosing care providers, breathing techniques, the labor process, and comfort measures. However, there is a deeper level of sacrifice that also shows up in labor that isn't addressed in childbirth preparation classes—the emotional and spiritual sacrifice of labor.

In the story of the Maiden Goddess, she must walk through seven Gates of Transformation, each requiring a sacrifice to cross the threshold, to complete her journey into the Underworld and become a mother. As birthing women, we too must walk through the same gates, not only to become a mother, but also to give our baby the gift of a lifetime— the chance at a healthy and optimal emotional foundation—because how we walk through these gates also affects our future child's psychology.

Science is confirming that psychological programming in humans is passed down through the generations in DNA[3]. That means that the unborn baby "marinates" inside amniotic fluid flavored with the emotional life and state of mind, as well as the beliefs, habits, addictions, and tendencies of its DNA lineage (mom, grandparents, and great grandparents). For better or worse, the emotional state of the mother in pregnancy imprints on a baby's future sense of safety, self-worth, empathy, belonging, and capacity to have healthy relationships.

If pregnancy hasn't been one big ball of bliss, don't worry! Birth gives us an amazing opportunity to heal any and all unhealthy emotional programs, habits, and behaviors *and* can change the baby's emotional baseline for the better. Labor asks us to use these Gates of Transformation as an effective psychological shortcut to reprogram our DNA before it is solidified into a baby's personality.

When we choose to willingly walk through each of the Gates of Transformation and healthily approach our emotions, we can transform fear, shame, control, pain, independence, disassociation, and victimization into joy, worthiness, trust, connection, embodiment, and empowered surrender. When we start to look at birth from this perspective, we realize how labor can heal not only the baby, but our lineage as well. Perhaps this is why women get to have this spiritual shortcut—because we are the Gatekeepers of humanity. Intentionally breaking the chains of any toxic programming and infusing new neural pathways of healthy and positive belief systems into our babies before they are born is truly how we can shift humanity on a collective scale.

Birth is a Spiritual Transformation

Walking through the Gates of Transformation also rewards us with a deep sense of empowerment and self-mastery through the healing of past emotional traumas and the pleasure of surrendering to a higher power. As we dance with the waves of contractions throughout labor, we can spiral further and further down into our own personal Underworld. There, we will be asked to face the darkest parts of ourselves, look them square in the eye, and decide to choose a healthier way forward. If we prepare properly in pregnancy and unpack personal blocks to the gates before labor begins, we will find ourselves more confident to utilize labor as a spiritual tool of conscious enlightenment.

From Maiden-to-Mother

Birth is a transformation from an old self into a new self. To help us better understand this shift in energy, we use two feminine archetypes from the Maiden Goddess story: the Maiden and the Mother.

No matter where we are in life, when we are pregnant, we embody the archetype of the Maiden, and after birth, we embody the archetype of the Mother. If you have other children, you are balancing both archetypes at the same time. The Maiden embodies freedom, innocence, and adventure. For first-time mothers, she is the part of ourselves that has never had the responsibility of nurturing, raising, or guiding the life of a child 24/7. Instead, we have the freedom to explore the world guided by our own desires, on our own timeline, and at our own pace. We are not tied down by another human being, and the only responsibility we have is to our own happiness. We are free to do as we please: sleep in, stay out late, and follow our own whims. We sacrifice only for the self. It is the embodiment of the free lifestyle before children. This Maiden energy can be a difficult thing to let go of as we will see in a story of mom-to-be, Amy, later in this chapter.

For second or multiple-time moms-to-be, the Maiden shows up a little differently because we have already been initiated into motherhood at least once before. However, we still return to our inner Maiden when we become pregnant again, and we have another opportunity to deepen into self-mastery of our emotional Underworld and upgrade our motherhood skills. We've probably learned many valuable lessons from the last child and have healed more than we realize, and we can bring that new wisdom to our next birth experience for the benefit of all our children. And just because we have journeyed into the Underworld once before and have risen anew, it won't make this experience any less emotional, difficult or sacrificial. It will not make the journey feel any more familiar or known. Each birth is unique and different, and we will still have to face sacrifices, this time deeper and more thorough, to become a greater version of our Mother-self.

Mother Archetype

The Mother archetype is the part of us that has learned and fully embraced the idea of complete sacrifice for another. We now understand on all levels that life is no longer about ourselves, but about fostering, nurturing, and guiding someone else—a child completely dependent on us for survival, love, nourishment, and support. We have moved from a place of detached independence to attached, healthy codependence. Mother energy is one of continual, daily, never-ending sacrifice, surrender, and service to our children over and over again. For this sacrifice, we are rewarded with deep connection, a fulfilling purpose, and a bond that cannot be experienced in any other way. Pregnancy and labor attempt to teach us about this level of sacrifice, should we be willing to learn.

Labor can bring fear to both new and second-time moms-to-be; however, if we intentionally surrender to the process with love, we can reap the benefits of that sacrifice—an empowered and fulfilling birth experience and a confident entry into motherhood. To do so, we must sacrifice everything that keeps us tied to the old version of ourselves through deep emotional, spiritual, and psychological surrender.

Once we have fully entered into our Mother-self, we can use the sacred postpartum time to integrate this huge transformation. In Chapter 9, we explore how to best use this time for emotional and spiritual integration. During postpartum, we can joyfully embrace the new version of ourselves while simultaneously grieving and honoring what we have lost—our maidenhood. We use the word "grieve" because the Maiden has indeed died—along with all our dreams, hopes, wishes, and desires that can only live in the Maiden. There is a very real loss that most of society often simply labels as "baby blues." But what is really happening is deep grief that needs space, time, and compassion to sort through, all while simultaneously feeling the joy, elation, and euphoria from having a new baby. No wonder this time can feel so confusing!

Death of the Maiden

Birth requires the ultimate sacrifice—death. This is because birth cannot exist without death. It is part of the ebb and flow and the balance of life; two equal forces pushing and pulling; creating and destroying. There cannot be one without the other.

If we look around at our world, all we see is polarity—yin and yang, feminine and masculine positive and negative, night and day, spring and fall, up and down. Nothing lasts forever. Everything must transform at some point, and we are no different. And this can seem like a really scary prospect. This idea of death brings up fears around the loss of who we know ourselves to be and who we may become. It is an identity crisis of sorts.

But, the truth about Maiden death is that it is actually not really death at all—though it 100 percent feels like it. It is actually a transformation, a transition, a focused shift. Just like Mother Nature, nothing truly dies. If we understand our loss as a transformation into a more elevated expression rather than a disappearance, we can more easily move through the baby blues time of postpartum. This doesn't mean that we won't miss who we used to be or the freedom that we used to have—nostalgia will always be there. But if we can frame the transition as an evolution of the self, a building block that needs to be shifted, we find ourselves productively dealing with the grief.

A DOULA'S BIRTH STORY

Amy, a 33-year-old mother-to-be from New York City, described her journey as follows:

"A few months into the pregnancy, I hired a doula. We started prepping for all the physical aspects of my labor. After a prenatal visit, it hit me . . . I'm going to be a MOM! Oh, my God! I have to give up everything! Who I am. What I am. How I live my life! This revelation scared the crap out of me. Intellectually, I knew life was going to be different, and I thought I was okay with that, but what I didn't understand was how my essence, my core being, was going to change. I completely broke down."

> Using the Gates of Transformation of the Maiden Goddess metaphor during pregnancy, Amy was able to come to terms with the death of her Maiden-self and fully transform, but it was difficult. For her, the most challenging part was the realization that a part of her had to die, so a new, higher aspect could be born. The point of sharing this story is that sometimes the hardest thing to do is acknowledge and honor the mini-deaths, and the ultimate death of the Maiden, as a sacrifice for motherhood. Knowing what will occur and accepting it for what it is—not just a death, but a rebirth—really helped Amy move through it all.
>
> **As witnessed by Lauren Mahana**

In this story, Amy had a sudden recognition that her pending sacrifice was daunting, and it felt exhausting. Amy knew she had to transform, but the real struggle was the sacrifice, and it brought up questions like:

- If I give this up, what else do I have to give up?
- When I sacrifice this aspect, do I completely lose myself?
- Am I no longer me?

These questions are completely valid, normal, and natural. They might stir up some fear of the unknown. The very idea that we must trust a sacrifice as a tool for expansion is terrifying. How can these questions be answered with truthful knowledge? This is the journey of the Maiden Goddess, the Gates of Transformation, and this book.

We Can't Avoid Sacrifice in Birth

We might be tempted to ask, "How can I get through these gates unscathed or without sacrifice?" The answer is, we can't. If we want to become mothers, then the gates will show up, and sacrifices will be required. *How* we sacrifice at each of the gates will make or break us. We have two choices in how: willingly with empowerment, or unwillingly with pain and resistance. Our actions and reactions to our sacrifices are completely up to us. In fact, it is really the only thing we have total control over in birth!

So, what happens when we don't walk through the gates freely and willingly? Well, we can end up getting dragged through them because, as we said, we can't escape sacrifice. We will have to do it one way or another. When we resist, we run the risk of getting ourselves psychologically stuck in that moment of fearful stubbornness and resistance. Unfortunately, this unwillingness can and does lead to emotional trauma, victimization, shame, and regret in the birth experience—all feelings of a disempowered birth. These are the exact experiences that we hope to avoid, by showing you the healthy, healing techniques laid out at each gate in the coming chapters. Understanding that resistance is only going to cause pain is hopefully motivation enough to dive into each sacrifice with an open heart and mind.

Motherhood is the definition of sacrifice. Every day when we wake up next to baby, we are sacrificing our own freedom, individuality, sleep, comfort, energy, and emotions all in the name of another's benefit. We have entered into a brand-new way of being that is all about serving someone else. We learn it is much easier to navigate this new way of life if we willingly sacrifice what is necessary, not what is easy. By accepting this truth, we set ourselves up to walk through the gates with grace and honor. So, why not take the Maiden Goddess's lead and lean into the sacrifice? Why resist when we can assist in our own personal transformations?

As we navigate the different levels of sacrifice of pregnancy and labor, we are encouraged to continually come back to the idea that "mother" is a Divine sacrifice of love. That is the essence of the energy we are each becoming. The hope is that we learn the habit of surrendering to the necessary sacrifices and lessons that each of the Gates of Transformation wants to teach us with grace, empowerment, and strength of character.

The Gates of Transformation

The rest of the chapters in this book take you through each of the Gates of Transformation, step by step. You will learn how to:

- Recognize each gate as it shows up in your own pregnancy and labor
- Learn to process any emotions or traumas that may keep you from fully surrendering to any and all of the Gates of Transformation
- Surrender to each sacrifice with willingness, empowerment, and love
- Integrate a new reality of thinking and feeling using the provided Integration Practices

The following chart offers an overview of the seven gates with the metaphorical and actual sacrifices as well as the rewards you will reap once you move through the gate.

GATES OF TRANSFORMATION

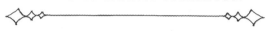

GATE	METAPHORICAL SACRIFICE	PSYCHOLOGICAL SACRIFICE	EMOTIONAL SACRIFICE	REWARD
Gate of Courage and Sovereignty	Sword	Overcoming old ways of coping with fear	Facing fear	Courage, sovereignty, empowerment
Gate of Vulnerability	Cloak	Allowing yourself to be vulnerable	Owning unresolved shame and victimization	Self love, inner strength and self-acceptance
Gate of Expectations	Map	Releasing the need/desire to control	Letting go of mistrust- healing trauma	Trust in yourself and the divine, true faith
Gate of Embodiment	Locket	Letting go of desire to escape, numb, avoid or disassociate	Allowing yourself to feel all the feelings and sacrifices	True presence, embodiment, greater sovereignty
Gate of Sacred Partnership	Ability to walk	Giving up independence or doing things on your own	Putting aside the ego and grieving the maiden self as individual	Community, support, and the power of true partnership
Gate of Fortitude	Shoes	Reframing pain in your mind and removing self-sabotage	Feeling physical and emotional discomfort and pain	Patience, perserverance and inner fortitude
Gate of Intentional Surrender	Death	Releasing who you thought you were, ego death, spiritual death	Grieving the old self, feelings of loss, surrender	Your divine initiation into Motherhood

Each gate we cross deepens self-awareness and serves as a calling to become more expanded and healed versions of ourselves. These are the emotional hurdles that we must all move through to experience a fully embodied goddess birth. Each gate corresponds to a different metaphorical sacrifice that the Maiden Goddess in our story must also experience. At the end of the story, she realizes that she can never have become a mother without those sacrifices that allow her to fully embrace her transition into motherhood. As laboring women, we also understand that the sacrifices we make pave the way for the rewards we seek.

Another interesting thing to note about this journey is that each gate unlocks pain or stuck energy in a different part of the energetic chakra system. There are seven chakras (energy centers) through which our life force flows up the middle of our bodies, starting at our perineum and ending at our crowns. Each chakra holds a different set of energetic information as it relates to our lives, and as we go through each gate, that corresponding chakra is activated and healed. For example, the first chakra (located at our perineum) holds information about survival, fight-flight-freeze, primal instinct, security, money, and safety. The first chakra is where we store our fears. The purpose of each of the Gates of Transformation is to unlock and heal the chakras. For example, the Gate of Courage and Sovereignty unlocks the energy in the first chakra and activates our fear so we can face and heal it as we cross over the threshold. As the chart below shows, each gate gives us energetic healing as we initiate ourselves emotionally into motherhood. This is what makes this process so powerful.

These chakras show us where emotional blockages can occur within the mind, body, and soul when we labor. The gates acknowledge that energy doesn't always flow freely and purposefully but often needs to be worked through. Emotional and energetic stagnation must be brought into awareness to transform, and this is exactly what each gate offers us. As we move through the labor journey, we understand firsthand this correspondence and synchronicity between the seven gates and the seven chakras.

If you practice yoga or meditation, you're probably familiar with the chakras. If not, here follows a summary of the name and system:

THE CHAKRA SYSTEM

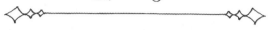

CHAKRA NAME	LOCATION ON THE BODY	THEME OF THE CHAKRA	EMOTIONS IN THE CHAKRA	CORRESPONDING GATE
First: Root and support chakra (Muladhara)	Perineum	Survival, security, instinct, safety	Fear, anxiety, fight/flight response	Gate of Courage and Sovereignty
Second: Sensual and emotional chakra (Svadhisthana)	Womb	Creativity, sexuality, feminine connection	Shame, self-worth, sensuality, creative power	Gate of Vulnerability
Third: Personal power chakra (Manipura)	Solar Plexus	Personal power, expectations, competition	Control, frustration, anger, desire to fight	Gate of Expectations
Fourth: Affinity chakra (Anahata)	Heart	Affinity, openness, compassion and presence	Inner joy, satisfaction, being present, fully feeling	Gate of Embodiment
Fifth: Self-expression chakra (Vishudha)	Throat	Speaking out, asking, questioning and voicing the truth	Fear of self-expression or asking for help, untruths	Gate of Sacred Partnership
Sixth: Third-eye chakra (Ajna)	Center of head, third-eye	Inner vision, psychic gifts, beliefs and thoughts	Neutrality, curiosity, validation, perserverance	Gate of Fortitude
Seventh: Crown chakra (Sahasrara)	Top of head, crown	Connection to spirit, inner divinity, transformation	Soul resonance, satisfaction, faith and inner knowing	Gate of Intentional Surrender

The theme of each chakra aligns with the sacrifice required to cross each of the seven Gates of Transformation, which further exemplifies them as portals of spiritual growth. If we replace the word "gate" with "chakra," we get a completely different experience of the Maiden Goddess journey. For example, the Maiden Goddess moves through the first chakra and sacrifices her sword, which for her represents her protection. Being able to see the connections between the gates and the chakras allows us to utilize the techniques in this book to heal. When we practice walking through these gates in pregnancy, we can learn where we might need additional support in the form of energy healing because we are aware of where the energy is stagnant. Another great reason to start this journey now.

How to Walk Through the Gates of Transformation

Each chapter for the rest of this book focuses on an individual Gate of Transformation, the themes of that gate, the symbolism in the Maiden Goddess story and the sacrifices that will be asked of you to cross over the threshold to walk through the gate. The simple willingness to explore each chapter with an open mind and open heart is a powerful step into your own emotional Underworld.

You may find, that as you read the chapters, some topics may feel more intense than others and elicit a physical or emotional reaction within you. This is actually a great thing! Your body is showing you where resistance currently lives that could possibly get you stuck at that gate when labor begins. Understanding your own resistance and what that looks like will show you what still needs to be healed on your journey from Maiden-to-Mother. So, look out for moments where you may hastily dismiss an idea presented or feel triggered, angry, or upset. These emotional signposts are your resistance telling you there is deeper work to be uncovered here.

As this happens, you may find yourself needing deeper support to work through the resistance to the gate or the sacrifices required. In these instances, we've developed four different types of Integration Practices, which have worked successfully with our clients, at the end of each chapter, as follows:

- *SELF-LOVE ACTIVITIES* to help you find fierce compassion and love for yourself as you move through the Gates of Transformation. It's very easy when we are in resistance to a gate or sacrifice to leave behind self-love in place of self-judgment. These activities are created to cultivate and return to the energy of love needed to break through resistance.

- *INNER EXPLORATION JOURNAL PROMPTS* to help you dive deep into your own emotional Underworld and discover realities within yourself that may be unknown to you. The act of writing gives a voice to the inner parts of yourself that have been silenced, traumatized, scared, or ignored over the years. Each prompt asks direct and powerful questions to draw out possible emotional blocks that can trip you up in labor.

- *GODDESS RITUALS* to help you connect more deeply with Divine Feminine Energy, the intention of your birth, and the spiritual nature of your transition from Maiden-to-Mother. These are great practices if you find the spiritual aspects we talk about challenging or foreign. Each ritual is designed to help you integrate the lessons of each gate, so they become part of a new reality before labor begins.

- *THRESHOLD MEDITATIONS* to help you visualize your personal crossing of the threshold of each Gate of Transformation, especially when resistance is strong. Meditation is a powerful and effective way to prepare the mind for such a transition as well as quiet or calm the parts of the mind that want to avoid change. Meditation is a practical way to rewire our minds to be more supportive.

Because each journey through birth is so different, it is important to let your intuition guide you through these practices. Take your time, and do the ones that speak to your heart. Give yourself space to reflect, and you will find integration enjoyable and enlightening. And, of course, please reach out to a professional therapist, healer, or counselor should you need additional support to walk through each Gate of Transformation with empowerment.

Before we begin this deep journey into the Underworld to become mothers, we highly recommend taking time to explore these first Integration Practices. The following are meant to help find your emotional, spiritual, and psychological baseline before starting on the journey of this book. You'll experience so much transformation over the next eight chapters (and throughout your pregnancy), that it is a good idea to know where you are at the beginning. Think of it as a "before" snapshot to help you quantify your transformation when you finish this book. If this resonates with you and your process, please enjoy the following practices:

Integration Practices

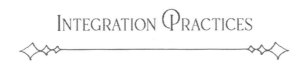

What is more of a beginning than your own birth story? Learning how you were born into the world can give you a lot of insight into the struggles, lessons, and challenges that you have faced up until now and that may show up when you start to walk through the gates. The energy that was in your own mother's womb was the marinade you soaked in for nine months, setting your personality and emotional foundations, so let's explore the energy that made you.

Self-Love Activity: Discover Your Birth Story

In this exercise, we invite you to reach out to the people who were witnesses at your birth (mother, father, grandparents, aunts/uncles, family friends, and so on) or those who may have heard your birth story. Ask the witnesses or yourself the questions below. You want to figure out how you were welcomed into the world and what the circumstances were around your birth that created your own personal foundation of safety, self-worth, and belonging. If you're unable to reach out to anyone, try to remember what you can from what you know about your own birth.

- What time did labor start? Where was your mother? What was she doing?
- What was happening in the world on that day? What was the weather like?
- What kind of birth was it? Painful? Beautiful? Fast? Slow? Traumatic? Scary?
- Who was present for the birth? Where did it happen?
- How long did your mother labor? How long did she push?
- Did you breastfeed? If so, did you latch easily?

- How did she feel throughout the birth? How did she feel once you were born?
- What did she say while in labor? What did she say once you were born?

Try to find the true essence of that day, the space, and how it felt for all who witnessed. Talk to the different witnesses on their own so you can understand their individual points of view. If you were adopted or are unable to speak with any witnesses of your birth, you may want to see a spiritual healer who can help you discover your birth story through meditation, shamanic healing, or past-life regression. See Recommended Resources at the back of the book.

INNER EXPLORATION JOURNAL PROMPTS

Once you have heard the perspective of a birth witness, write it down and begin to answer the following journal prompts:

- How does my birth story make me feel?
- Does my birth story make sense as it relates to my life experience?
- Does my birth story set the tone for my challenges and lessons in life? If so, how?
- Do I still carry the weight of my birth?
- How has my birth experience affected my relationship with my mother? Did it bring us closer or further apart?
- Do I want my child's birth to be similar or completely different?

Now start to focus on how you may or may not have been feeling when you were a tiny baby making her entrance into the world. Use your imagination to answer these questions:

- How did it feel to be birthed in this way as a baby?
- Did my birth feel empowering or disempowering to my baby self?
- What feelings may have come up for me as a baby after this birth experience?
- As a baby, how did I feel about my birth, my mother, and my father?

- Did my birth allow for me to go at my own pace, or was I rushed or pushed in some way?
- Has this affected my relationship currently with accepting my own rhythm?

Now, focus on the idea of healing any parts of your birth story or yourself that feel broken or wounded. Ask yourself:

- What needs to be healed, so my baby doesn't have to carry extra burdens?
- What birth trauma needs to be processed before I go into labor?
- How can I heal my womb space by healing my own birth?
- What programming that I know is in my DNA do I not want to pass on to my baby?
- What habits or behaviors do I not want to pass on to my baby?
- What can I do now and in labor to be conscious of this programming as it shows up?

This is just the beginning of your deep journey into self-discovery, and you can build upon this journal entry through each gate. If you are fortunate enough to have a living grandparent, you might wish to take this entire exercise to a previous generation. Ask them about the birth of your parents. Ask the same questions you did about your own birth. Write it all down. You might even want to record your elder. This is something that you can share with your child later in life.

After you finish your conversations and hear the various stories, look for similarities and differences. Can you see a pattern of word choice or events? The point of this exercise is to identify any recurring traumas or noticeable healings that happened in labor in your lineage. This is the beginning of your exploration of your spiritual and genetic lineage. Not only will this allow you to see the storylines, themes, and common struggles, you will also be able to extrapolate and connect cultural and ethnic traumas. This will lead you down an intensely beautiful collective healing for your ancestors and future generations.

__Bonus__

Do this exercise for your partner's side of the family as well. Help your partner move through their own birth story so that they too can be healed before labor begins.

GODDESS RITUAL: CREATE A BIRTH ALTAR

Just like the Maiden Goddess, you will walk through the Gates of Transformation to master your inner Maiden and transform into Mother. As you approach each gate, it is important to have a reference point, a reminder of why you are completing this journey, for the times when doubt or resistance arises. For the Maiden Goddess, her statement of "I long to become a mother" is enough to remind her to continue her way forward, despite sacrifice and challenge.

However, the Maiden Goddess has the advantage of moving through the gates without distraction. We don't get the same benefit. Modern life, work, family, and everyday obligations can confuse our focus and make us forget our intentions for our pregnancy and labor. This is why creating a birth altar can help direct your focus while working through each gate in pregnancy. An altar is a special space that you set aside as a sacred spot in your home to hold your intention and a reminder for times of uncertainty. It can be a corner of your home or the place you choose to read this book. It doesn't need to be large or elaborate. All you need is a small flat space where you can place meaningful objects, letters, crystals, statues, images, or anything else that reminds you of your birth intention. Place things that invoke a strong sense of love, joy, and empowerment around your conception, your birth, and your family.

Some of you mamas may want to follow the rules of altar creation; others will just want to wing it and allow intuition to guide you. This is *your* journey!

If you need inspiration, here follows a list of objects that correlate with birth that you may like to place on your altar:

BIRTH ALTAR IDEAS

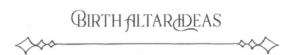

SACRED OBJECTS	CRYSTALS ASSOCIATED WITH BIRTH
Find objects that spark joy and excitement within you when you see them, touch them, smell them, etc., for example: • Images of your ancestors • Sonogram picture of your baby • Images of pomegranates or seedlings • Chalice or cup to represent your womb • Wand or staff to represent masculine energy • Vision board for your future family and birth experience	Focus on crystals that help the heart and womb chakras. Stones that help with grounding anxiety and stress, such as: • Unakite • Rhodochrosite • Rose quartz • Carnelian • Moonstone • Quartz • Lolite • Jade • Fluorite • Garnet
FERTILITY DEITIES	**COLORS AND SCENTS**
Find things that represent the divine energies of fertility, motherhood, fatherhood, pregnancy and birth like: • Demeter • Mother Mary • Artemis • Mary Magdalene • Oshun • Freya • Isis • Brigid • Hathor • Hera • Juno	Using colored candles and adorning them with particular scents can be very powerful way to honor your altar. Use these: • Green • Rose Oil • Red • Ylang Ylang Oil • Pink • Frankincesse Oil • Violet • Myrrh Oil • White • Mugwort Oil • Gold

Final Thoughts

It's now time to embark on your own journey from Maiden-to-Mother through the seven Gates of Transformation. Are you ready to start this grand adventure? We will be with you every step of the way as you learn about the gates, the sacrifices, and the rewards that await. Take your time and allow the wisdom of each chapter to unlock deeper layers of self-knowing, inner trust, and empowerment for both you and your baby. You are a Divine birth goddess in the making!

~ CHAPTER II ~

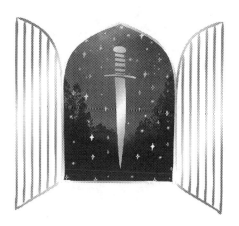

THE GATE OF COURAGE AND SOVEREIGNTY

OVERCOMING FEAR

You can choose courage, or you can choose comfort, but you can't choose both.

—*Brene Brown*

She left the meadow that she called home and began down the dark path into the Underworld. Her heart was beating loudly, and she jumped at every noise of the night. She reassured herself that with her sword by her side, she would be safe.

After a few hours of walking in darkness, she approached the first of many gates that she had been warned she would need to walk through. This first gate was made of iron, large and standing in the middle of the forest. It was enchanted with magic, so even though it looked like you could just walk around it, an invisible wall blocked the way. The Maiden Goddess quickly realized that the only way to get past this gate was to figure out how to walk through it. So, she decided to knock. She knocked, and knocked, and knocked, hoping someone would answer.

Finally, an old hag Gatekeeper appeared, asking the Maiden Goddess what business she had knocking on her door. She boldly and bravely replied, "I long to become a mother. I am on my way to the Underworld."

"Ah, yes, I see," said the Gatekeeper. "You can only get there through me. You must walk through this gate, but the only way I will let you through is if you give me something as a sacrifice in return." The Maiden Goddess kicked herself for not bringing any gold to pay this old crone for passage.

"I have no money—" said the Maiden Goddess.

"I don't want your money, dear Maiden. No, I think I'll take that sword you have on your hip, and I will allow you to continue to the Underworld." The Gatekeeper sneered.

"My sword! But how will I protect myself without it? The journey to the Underworld is dangerous, even if I am a goddess. I'm going to need it to keep myself safe. There must be something else I can give you instead."

The Gatekeeper replied, "The sword, Maiden Goddess. This is the sacrifice required. You will just have to learn to face your fears without a sword to protect you."

The Maiden Goddess thought about this impossible request, turning over different scenarios in her mind. How she could possibly survive the journey without it? But the inner calling to become a mother urged her to sacrifice her sword, despite logic begging her to turn around.

With hesitation, reluctance, and fear, she handed over the sword to the Gatekeeper, and the iron gates flung open. Endless darkness was all she could see in front of her, and the fear of what could be out there struck her heart and froze every muscle in her body. She found herself unable to cross the threshold.

After some time staring her fear in the face, she summoned the strength to say to herself, "I will not be afraid of the darkness, and I will not be a slave to my fears. I am safe without my sword, and I am full of courage. I will walk through this gate with a crown of sovereignty upon my head and my heart."

Her fears melted into motivation, and she bravely crossed the gate into the darkness of the Underworld.

Fear and the First Gate

Fear—that dreaded four-letter word—can either save us or crush us as mothers. For many reasons, fear and childbirth seem inseparable. From the moment we conceive our babies, we worry about their health, their growth, their gestation, the foods we eat, the sensations we feel, and so on, and so forth. When we go into labor, we fear the pain of contractions, the length and intensity of labor, and being vulnerable to our caregivers. Parenting is no different. We fear whether or not our kids are safe, happy, well-adjusted, independent, and compassionate people. It seems we just can't escape fear as mothers. And that's okay.

Not all fear is bad—a little can actually be a positive, useful, and powerful tool when, for example, we need to protect our children. But, left unchecked, fear has the habit of poisoning our mental wellbeing and negatively affecting our ability to parent from trust and love. How fear manifests is determined by *how* we face our fears. Do we do so with courage and sovereignty? Or do we choose to avoid, hide from, or numb ourselves to them? Facing our fears as mothers rather than maidens is the first lesson we must learn as we move into motherhood and is the first offering of sacrifice on our journey into the Underworld.

In our story, the Maiden Goddess learns that handling her fear empowers her transition into motherhood. She must sacrifice her sword (a.k.a., the old, perhaps unhealthy ways, she has avoided her fears in the past) and find her inner courage (the strength to act in spite of fear) to walk through the gate and conquer her fears with true sovereignty. As pregnant women, we must also do the same: empower ourselves and set a strong foundation for our motherhood.

Healthy Fear vs. Unhealthy Fear

To ensure a smooth transition, we first need to recognize the difference between healthy fear and unhealthy fear. Let's talk about healthy fear first.

Healthy fear is the fear of danger that is in real-time, in real-life, and needed to survive a present threat. There is often an intuitive and "street-smart" quality to healthy fear that keeps us safe and aware. This is the kind of fear that tells us to not walk down a dark alley in a bad neighborhood or eat those moldy leftovers. Healthy fear heightens our awareness of our surroundings, keeps our behavior in check, and improves our ability to react effectively to dangerous situations.

In pregnancy, we face healthy fear almost daily as we take care of our bodies for our babies. The very healthy fear of fetal birth defects prevents most of us from indulging in booze and cigarettes or riding rollercoasters. Healthy fear can be a positive motivator for behavior necessary for survival, especially in an emergency situation. For example, imagine a pregnant woman whose water just broke and who finds herself running from a wild animal. Her healthy fear signals adrenaline to surge throughout her body, which will cause her labor to slow or stop completely until she reaches safety. This reaction keeps both mom and baby alive until a safer environment emerges so the baby can be born. It is in these emergency situations that adrenaline is helpful for the safe delivery of the baby. However, in a non-emergency birth, adrenaline is the last thing we want to show up.

But here is the thing about healthy fear: once the threat of danger has been eliminated, the fear disappears, the adrenaline fades, and our bodies return to a normal emotional equilibrium. This is because healthy fear lives only in the present moment. If there is no danger, then there is no fear. However, every so often, fear (and adrenaline) can linger long after the danger has gone, or they can pop up even where there is no present danger. This is an unhealthy fear.

Unhealthy fear is fear due to *perceived or imagined danger*, rather than actual danger. It is tricky because, in our minds, we believe that the danger is real and so behave accordingly. The longer we live with unhealthy fear, the greater the risk of losing touch with reality. Imagine the overprotective mother who won't let her children out of her sight because she believes that danger is lurking around every corner. Her world is tainted by unhealthy fear that probably started small and has snowballed over the years, because she never faced it and never walked through this gate. She resisted it, and her fear persisted when, in reality, the danger surrounding her children was very low. So, her perceived danger of allowing her children to play at a responsible neighbor's house or visit with grandparents without her watchful eye is irrational and purely emotional. But she cannot see this truth because she is so overcome with unhealthy fear. It stunts her ability to parent and help her children learn independence.

This is why unhealthy fear can be so dangerous: it starts as a little seed and grows exponentially if we don't face it with courage. This is another reason the wise crone Gatekeeper demands the Maiden Goddess to sacrifice her sword. The sacrifice allows the Maiden to release the unhealthy fears that keep her out of reality.

Staying Mindful of Fear

Unhealthy fear isn't rooted in the present, but is usually triggered by the past (like a traumatic event) or the future (like the chronic anxiety about something that may occur). Whenever our minds focus on the past or the future, we become susceptible to unhealthy fear. This is why staying in the present moment, especially in labor, is a great way to cultivate courage—it doesn't allow our minds to fall prey to unhealthy fear. (In Chapter 5 we will delve more deeply into how powerful being present can be in labor.) But this can be very difficult for a lot of women who use chronic worry as a way to feel safe and in control (see Chapter 4 on releasing control). When we worry about the future or fear that the past will return, we aren't actually dealing with our unhealthy fears, but rather being victimized by them, caught in a fear-loop that makes it difficult to break out of it. This is what the Gatekeeper understood could happen to the Maiden if she kept her sword. We too must sacrifice any addictions to stress, worry, anxiety, and fear if we want to move through this gate with courage and sovereignty.

It can be difficult to determine if we are in healthy fear or unhealthy fear, so asking a few questions can help you find clarity:

- Is the danger I perceive actually happening, or is it just something I am worried about?
- Is this fear in the present moment, or is it triggering something from the past or worry for the future?
- Am I facing my fears with courage, or am I running away from them?

Asking these three questions each time you experience fear during pregnancy, labor, and motherhood is a powerful way to distinguish between healthy and unhealthy fear. And when we know what we are dealing with, we can figure out how to face it.

A DOULA'S BIRTH STORY

Bobbie was a chronic worrier. Throughout her pregnancy, she was sick with fear about every "what if" around the baby that crossed her mind. These fears started to affect her wellbeing, her sleep, and her relationship with her partner—and even the baby. At 28 weeks, Bobbie's high stress level caused her to go into preterm labor. She was rushed to the emergency room and told that it was too soon for the baby to be born. All the fears she had worried about for months now came rushing into reality, and she went into a full-on panic attack. The doctor on-call informed her that if she couldn't calm down and give her labor a chance to stop, she was going to have her baby right then and there—which was Bobbie's worst nightmare.

So Bobbie called me, and together, we started to look at the fears that were showing up. After 20 minutes of honest introspection and lots of tears, Bobbie realized that she was deeply afraid of being a bad mother and felt unprepared for the experience. She actually didn't have any fear around the baby being born early and felt she could handle that scenario. The moment she had this realization and was able to identify her real fear, her contractions slowed down, and her labor stopped.

Bobbie had been using anxiety and worry as a way of avoiding what was truly scaring her. We joked together that her baby just wanted her to face her real fears, so he didn't have to sit in that stress anymore. Bobbie calmed down for the rest of her pregnancy and used the techniques in this book to face her fears of motherhood. She delivered a healthy baby boy at 42 weeks and was excited for this new chapter of life.

As witnessed by Alexandria Moran

Sacrificing Our Metaphorical Swords

Let's talk about the sacrifice of this gate—the metaphorical sword. We've touched briefly on the different meanings of the sword and why the Maiden Goddess must give it up. Now, let's dive a little deeper into the struggle both our Maiden Goddess and pregnant women have with this particular sacrifice, because it is not an easy one. Why do we have to give up protection and a sense of safety on the journey into motherhood? Well, the answer is threefold:

First, the tools that worked for us in the past were developed and created to support our Maiden-selves. As we transition into motherhood, we have to sacrifice much of our Maiden-selves, and this includes the tools we've accumulated. We need a new set of tools to support our new selves—our Mother-selves. In this gate, the tools we are sacrificing are our coping mechanisms—habits, beliefs around fear, sense of safety, avoidance of courage, lack of vulnerability, and old ways of protection. The ways we used to cope in the past won't prove useful to us anymore. As we saw in the story of Bobbie, her old coping mechanism of using anxiety and worry as a way of avoiding her true fears wasn't going to work in motherhood, and she needed to hand over that old "sword" to move through the gate. The tools of the Maiden have no place in our new lives as Mother.

Giving up our trusty coping mechanisms can make us feel vulnerable, especially if we don't know how to deal with our fears without them. We often don't trust that we can be courageous enough. This gate is asking us to understand that we are capable of more than we think and we need to start with a clean slate, so we can create a new set of tools founded in courage, trust, and sovereignty. We must be willing to release the old so we can learn a new way forward.

Second, these metaphorical swords give us a false sense of self-preservation and, in the process, hinder our ability to cultivate true inner strength and courage. Courage is the willingness to face danger, difficulty, uncertainty, and pain in spite of fear—not in the absence of it. It requires vulnerability, and hiding behind old self-protection mechanisms, like a sword, keeps us out of our vulnerability. Courage requires vulnerability or it isn't courage. So, in truth, any protection or coping mechanism we bring into labor is actually keeping us from walking through this gate, tethering us to our Maiden-selves, and preventing an empowered transition into motherhood.

Finally, just like the sword, most of our coping mechanisms are tools of war, meant to keep us protected and safe in a world of conflict. The sword is a weapon of war, not of love. It is forged with masculine aggression and defensiveness. As Maidens, we often had to protect ourselves from danger in a male-dominated world, so of course we needed an appropriate weapon to keep ourselves safe—a man's weapon. We learned masculine coping mechanisms that brought out our inner masculine strength as a means of survival. And it worked for maidenhood.

But motherhood is a different story. The masculine energy of war, conflict, protection, aggression, and defensiveness is the exact opposite energy than that which creates an empowered birth experience. Just think about what happens to the body when it is holding a sword and is ready to fight— it tightens, hardens, restricts, and contracts. Adrenaline pumps through the veins and puts us into a fight-flight-freeze response. We are prepared for a fight . . . for war.

But birth is not war. Birth is a divine, feminine act of surrender and love. We need all of our *feminine* energy of vulnerability present to birth our babies with courage. We need to be open, expand, stretch, surrender, and soften—physically, emotionally, mentally, and spiritually—into motherhood. We can't fight our way through it. So, in a very real sense, any masculine energy of protection in our bodies, minds, and birthplaces only hinders our natural feminine laboring abilities. As doulas, we have seen firsthand the devastating consequences when women bring war-energy into the birth room, from labor delays and birth complications, to a cascade of unwanted medical interventions. To prevent these difficult consequences, all we have to do is be willing to:

1. Acknowledge the metaphorical swords that keep us from facing our fears as embodied women and cultivating our inner courage; and
2. Leave them in the past.

The Maiden's Way

Most of us, before becoming mothers, might not have had the healthiest coping mechanisms for fear, danger, and creating a sense of inner security unless we've undergone a lot of therapy and introspection work. As Maidens, we aren't asked to face our fears, but rather "deal" with them, so we do just that. We learn to avoid our fear; pretend it doesn't exist; numb ourselves with food, drugs, or alcohol; lie to ourselves; and a number of other ways we learn to "get through" fear. Motherhood is a different story.

As we step into motherhood—and prepare the mind, body, and spirit for the incredible task of raising the next generation—we have to face our fears, look them straight in the eye, and cultivate the courage to act healthily in spite of them. This is no easy task, especially if we're not in the habit of doing so. Even in the story, the Maiden Goddess wrestles with the notion of facing her fears rather than hiding behind her sword. She has moments of doubt, fear, anxiety, and apprehension. But ultimately, she decides that her will to become a conscious and compassionate mother trumps any coping mechanism. So, with courage and sovereignty, she hands over her sword and walks through the gate with her head held high. In labor, we can have moments of doubt, fear, and apprehension too, but as long as we, too, choose to hand over what no longer serves us and wholeheartedly trust the unknown, we will walk through this gate with empowerment. However, we have to understand first what our fears are and where they come from.

The Collective Fear That Birth Is Dangerous

The greatest fear we face as pregnant women is the collective fear that childbirth is dangerous, scary, chaotic, life-threatening, painful, and unpredictable. For most of us, what we are taught about birth comes from the entertainment industry. We grow up seeing women screaming in agony on a gurney, being rushed down hospital hallways, always in an emergency situation, shouting at their partners and begging for drug relief from a physician. Birth is depicted as a fearful medical procedure that shouldn't even be attempted without a doctor. When we see or hear of stories of women giving birth at home, or unassisted, or God forbid, having an orgasmic birth experience, we might chalk them up to "fringe" outlier experiences, not the norm. *Everyone* knows that birth is anything but that.

We accept these depictions because the truth is most mamas-to-be have never actually witnessed a live birth before their own, so they are left to assume that it is how it's depicted in Hollywood. That is the biggest lie of all. As doulas, we've witnessed too many births to count, and what happens in the movies just simply doesn't happen in real life. In most cases, birth is actually a peaceful, slow, calm, intense, and empowering experience that gradually builds. Women laugh through their labors, kiss their partners, and sway with the rhythms of their bodies. They get breaks and sometimes even sleep through much of their labor. When left free to labor at their own pace, and in their own way, most births are rather physically and medically uneventful experiences and hugely transformative spiritual experiences.

Because most moms have never been in a birth room before their own, there is a lack of personal and experiential understanding of the natural birth process and the Gates of Transformation that every laboring woman experiences. So, when we arrive at our own birth, the spiritual, emotional, and psychological sacrifices can feel, well, overwhelming. If unprepared, we will use whatever coping tools (healthy or unhealthy) to get through it, just like we always have in the past and, in doing so, run the risk of resisting this Gate of Transformation. When we resist, we can get stuck in a fight-flight-freeze response, halting labor, or risking complications. Fear is natural in the birth room. It is *how we deal with the fear* that will decide whether or not we walk through this gate—the choice is always up to us.

When we lived in tribal communities, childbirth was just as much a part of life as basket weaving or cooking. All the women participated, and children witnessed birth from a young age. It was normal and exciting, and it created deep bonds among all who attended. When women grow up, seeing and supporting birth long before they give birth themselves, their full understanding of birth is more grounded, confident, and full of love. Fear didn't exist in the birth huts of our ancestors.

But these days, we can't even tell our children about the truth of birth because of this collective fear. We shield them from the normalcy of birth with fantasy stories of a stork that delivers miracles rather than showing them the true miracle of a woman transforming from her Maiden-self into her Mother-self. But why the hell would we tell our kids the truth, when we are so terrified of it?

This sentiment grows even stronger when we share fear-based stories of birth between ourselves as women. When we tell dramatic stories full of words like "emergency," "NICU," "no-pulse," and "not breathing," that provide even further evidence for ourselves and the collective that birth should be feared. This harmful thinking is so deeply rooted in our beliefs about birth that many women feel bad or wrong to speak about their perfectly healthy, beautiful, and yes, even orgasmic births. Normal or pleasurable birth gets demonized as "weird" because it doesn't fit the collective belief that birth is traumatic. And unfortunately, the women who have had beautiful, normal, peaceful, or orgasmic births stop sharing their experiences because they are looked at like something is wrong with them.

Facing and Overcoming Fear

As a pregnant woman, it is more important than ever to surround yourself with stories that are uplifting and paint the true picture of birth—a loving, positive, empowering, and peaceful process. This might mean saying "no" to movies that have chaotic birth scenes or excusing yourself gracefully when a group of women begins to share their horror-birth stories. You can love and support them after you have your baby, but there is just no need to put yourself in that energy while pregnant and preparing for your own Gates of Transformation.

The same goes for your actual labor process. Should someone bring fear energy into your space, it is your right as a laboring mother to excuse that practitioner, nurse, or even a family member from your birth. This is the first way we face our fears: by choosing what energy we will surround ourselves with so we can ensure we stay in that open and soft intention. Any energy that causes you to feel like you need to bring in your metaphorical sword to protect yourself should be removed immediately. Your partner can be a great asset in helping to establish this dynamic, and we will talk about this at length in Chapter 6.

Finally, the last thing that has created this collective fear of childbirth is the one thing that is meant to squelch said fear—the advancement of technology. Birthing technology has grown by leaps and bounds over the last 100 years, and many advancements have made birth much safer in emergency situations. In that respect, we have definitely minimized fear of maternal or infant death when lives are on the line. However, in normal, non-emergency birth, maternal and infant death rates are on the rise. What gives?

Technology has become a catch-22 in terms of addressing the collective fear around birth. In our modern-day society, babies don't technically need to be "labored" to be born into the world. With the advent of C-sections, inductions, Pitocin (a chemical used to mimic natural Oxytocin and cause uterine contractions), and vaginal extraction tools, a doctor can literally birth a baby into the world with little or no participation from the mother and little or no respect for the baby's timing. These tools that were designed to save lives have now become more and more routine. For example, C-section rates have soared and become more common in non-emergency situations, leaving many women feeling uninvolved in their birth experiences and feeling robbed of the opportunity to walk through their Gates of Transformation.

We really wish this was not the case, and in most situations, it is not, but it is important to understand the reality that birth is Big Business. The more interventions, the more the hospital can bill. Most laboring mothers want to take their time in labor unless a doctor advises otherwise. The biggest manipulative tool a medical professional can use is to make the mama believe that her baby is in danger when it really is not. This is the invoking of unhealthy fear and an important reason to choose a compassionate and patient medical team who is willing to put your emotional and physical needs above finances or convenience. Having strong communication with your birth team will help ensure that your birth space stays fear-free, and if you need help doing this, please see Chapter 4, the Gate of Expectations.

As you unpack the impact of the collective fear on your own story and uncover your own fears with the Integration Practices at the end of this chapter, ask yourself how you can infuse more courage into your pregnancy and your birth space. As doulas, we encourage families to start watching empowering, calm birth videos as a way of retraining the brain to see birth as a beautiful and courageous journey into motherhood. On our website, www.laborlikeagoddess.com, you'll find a list of our favorite empowering birth videos.

The Fear of Going Within

We can't talk about fear without talking about the fear of going within. The Maiden Goddess must travel to the Underworld to become a mother, and we too must travel into our own emotional and psychological Underworlds. That means we must be willing to go into our subconscious, dive into the unknown, and allow ourselves to be transformed by it.

Whenever we go into an unknown in any circumstance, it is human nature for a certain level of fear to show up—the unknown is scary. It's the premise of most horror movies. However, this fear of the unknown can keep us from exploring and integrating our fears around birth, thus allowing unhealthy fears to fester. And with our own subconscious, there can be a belief that if we start to really look at our fears (like the fear of pain in childbirth, tearing during pushing, or having a C-section, for example) we worry it will manifest what we don't want into reality. We can be afraid that putting any energy toward overcoming our fears will bring them into existence, so we often ignore them. The opposite is true.

The moment we acknowledge our fears, even voice them to another, is the moment we take back our power. The fear might still be there, but we are no longer victims to it. We regain our sovereignty. Just like the Maiden Goddess, we proclaim to ourselves, "No. No, I will not be afraid of the darkness, and I will not be a slave to my fears. I am safe, and I am brave. I will walk through this gate with a crown of courage upon my head and heart."

The moment we shine the light on the dark parts of ourselves is the moment we are healed. Awareness brings sovereignty, transformation, and choice. The courageous act of going within and acknowledging our fears is actually the most empowering thing we can do for ourselves in birth and can help release any resistance to our own emotional Underworlds. We can't fight the Gates of Transformation. We must surrender to them. The Integration Practices at the end of this chapter can help you move through any resistance to going within.

The Fear–Pain Cycle

If that isn't enough reason to convince you to go within and face your fears, consider the fear–pain cycle phenomenon, which states that the more fear that exists within a mother while she labors, the more she experiences her own physical sensations in birth as pain. New research shows that more fear equals more pain[4]. It is scientifically proven.

In contrast, the more trust a mother has while she labors, the more she experiences her birth as pleasurable. It's this level of courage and trust that makes it possible for women to have an "ecstatic" or "orgasmic" birth experience. As doulas, we have seen it happen more often than is reported, as it is the more natural energy of birth. Fear seems to be the unnatural energy, which is why some women experience so much more pain than others.

We go into great depths about pain in Chapter 7, but here we want to talk about how fear can affect the perception of pain in the brain. Fear isn't just an emotional or psychological experience, but a hormonal one too. Fear kicks our sympathetic nervous system into gear, altering our bodies to be in fight-flight-freeze response. Muscles tense and adrenaline (a doula's nemesis in birth) skyrockets dramatically, increasing a laboring woman's pain sensitivity. What's worse, adrenaline can take hours to process out of the body, so doulas try to keep it out of the equation if at all possible. Enduring hours of heightened pain sensitivity due to a fear reaction is a laboring woman's worst nightmare.

Sacrificing our metaphorical swords helps keep adrenaline low and our pain threshold manageable. What we really want in birth is for oxytocin to flood our systems, and this amazing love molecule only shows up when we are relaxed, in love, and in total trust. This is why most "natural laboring techniques" emphasize relaxation as a pain deterrent. Oxytocin is the hormone released when we have an orgasm or eat a delicious chocolate cake, for example. It signals to our brains to shift into the parasympathetic mode (rest and restore) which is where we want to be operating from when we are laboring.

One of the best ways to break free of the fear–pain cycle is to focus on creating love and trust in the birth environment. We go into greater depths on how to do this in Chapters 4 and 5, but in the meantime, just know that all you really need to do is help yourself feel good while in the throes of contractions. Take a relaxing shower, self-pleasure, kiss your life-partner, cuddle a loved one or a pet, listen to soothing music, or allow yourself to be massaged. Surrender and soften. This will help calm that fear–pain cascade and bring back your sovereignty over your own pain.

The Reward of Courage and Sovereignty

With great sacrifice comes great reward. The journey to motherhood is no different. The Maiden Goddess sacrifices her old emotional and physical coping mechanisms but is rewarded with something even more valuable: true courage and sovereignty. She is fortified and empowered in her own ability to face her fears on the journey and doesn't end up missing her sword one bit.

So, what is sovereignty? Sovereignty is the freedom to act, feel, and believe as we wish without external control or subconscious sabotage. In the case of this gate, the Maiden Goddess frees herself from the control of her own unhealthy fears and coping mechanisms through the power of courage. Courage begets sovereignty. Sovereignty feeds our trust in courage. The more courage we cultivate, the more sovereignty we feel, and the more courage we have when we really need it. This is truly the recipe for empowerment.

However, when we are faced with fear and feel helpless or vulnerable, it is very easy to give sovereignty over to the nearest authority figure as an attempt to feel safe again in a moment of uncertainty. It's like we are saying to ourselves, "OMG. . . I can't handle this . . . You there, you make the call for me. I trust you more than I trust myself." This is a dangerous situation for any laboring mother to get herself into, and sometimes we start this habit in pregnancy, even before we begin the journey into the Underworld, with our doctors and family members.

The number-one regret we hear from moms in postpartum support groups about their labor is that they felt that someone else (a family member, a partner, a doula, or a medical professional) made decisions on their behalf and that they weren't in control of their own agency when they were at their most vulnerable state in labor. This causes a lot of emotional suffering, guilt, resentment, and confusion in moms trying to piece together how certain decisions were made when labor seems like a haze in hindsight. Some moms even have PTSD (post-traumatic stress disorder) because of this lack of sovereignty, self-agency, and boundaries.

As women, it isn't always easy to speak up when our boundaries are crossed. It's even harder when we are at our most vulnerable and exhausted from labor. Now, add an authoritarian figure saying scary things and pressuring us—and we can forget about any self-sovereignty. That is, unless we are practiced in it.

But most of us aren't naturals at self-sovereignty and we often place medical professionals on a pedestal of authority because we assume they know more than us. Many moms-to-be will allow a doctor's opinion to trump her own because of an assumed level of authority or knowledge.

This is partially due to what's known as the "White Lab Coat" effect—a phenomenon in which a white lab coat automatically elevates a person's credibility and authority whether or not they are qualified or have truthful information. As doulas, we've seen nurses and doctors unconsciously say things that were medically incorrect just to get a laboring woman to do what they wanted—usually, to hurry up labor. Because of their perceived level of authority over the laboring woman, the woman usually agrees. Many times, this works out in the end, but it can also make a woman feel slighted and disempowered, even though, at the time, she was happy to do what the nurse/doctor suggested. Relying on medicine or doctors to feel safe is just another coping mechanism that can keep us from handing over the proverbial sword and facing our fears. But the inner emotional abandonment that happens as a result of it can cause a lot of postpartum memory trauma and leave some new moms lacking confidence in their ability to speak up for themselves.

Later in this chapter, we will take you through some Integration Practices to develop the skills needed to maintain sovereignty while facing your fears, so you can have an empowered birth experience. If you find you struggle with inner agency with authority figures, start to practice the skills taught now because incorporating these habits in your everyday life will set you up for success when you are in the throes of labor.

It is important to note that most medical professionals are extremely sensitive to agency and will take their time to explain things as much as you'd like, if you ask. If they aren't willing to support you in this way, you may want to find another team—one that respects your sovereignty and makes it their goal for you to feel empowered about all medical decisions. But it is up to you to assume that self-responsibility, ask the important questions, take the time you need to make decisions, and tune in with your own intuition. Only then will your sovereignty reign.

How to Walk Through the Gate of Courage and Sovereignty

Much of this chapter is about the challenges of this gate, but how exactly do you hand over your metaphorical sword so you can walk through this gate and receive the blessings of courage and sovereignty?

As we've already mentioned and alluded to earlier, the first step is to bring your fears into your awareness. If you've been knee-deep in maidenhood, you've probably never even given your fears a chance to be seen or heard. Why would you? It's scary in there.

This gate is going to ask you to take a deep dive into your own emotional Underworld, to dig up your fears and acknowledge their existence. Using the following journal prompts and Integration Practices, you will be able to really explore any hidden fears that might be waiting to pop up the moment you go into labor.

Once you have identified your fears, you will need to notice where your metaphorical sword (a.k.a., your coping mechanisms) shows up and prevents you from feeling your fears and being vulnerable. Perhaps you use avoidance swords, like food, TV, sex, or total denial to numb yourself to fear. Or perhaps you swing in the opposite direction and go full control-freak in developing a Plan B, Plan C, Plan D, and Plan Z as your metaphorical sword. Acknowledging where your daily habits rely on your sword can start to give you sovereignty from them. When you see how much you rely on old forms of protection and self-preservation, you can start to make different moves or, better yet, just face the fears, so you no longer need a sword.

Finally, once you know your fears and metaphorical swords, it's time to hand them over to the Gatekeeper. This can be more of a process than a moment. Sometimes it might take you a little longer to fully let go of your safety net; other times you'll know you're done with them and just release them immediately. Each time you go through this gate, it will be different. Cultivating compassion and understanding for yourself during this process is key. The more self-love you feel, the more you will be able to teach your baby how to emotionally take care of and love themselves. It's a powerful process that takes time . . . so let yourself have it!

The best way to hand over your sword is by creating a safe, *threshold moment.* In our story, the Maiden Goddess crosses the gate's threshold as a way of truly stepping into her courage and sovereignty while leaving behind her fears. You can do the same on a more energetic level. Threshold moments can be any moment you express or verbalize your fears to another person you trust. This act of acknowledgment can be cathartic and healing on many levels. Another way to create a threshold moment is to design a personal ritual ceremony, where you can walk across a threshold as a symbolic release of the old ways. This is a powerful self-initiation rite that many pregnant mamas find very helpful in their own journeys as it combines the physical, spiritual, and emotional aspects in one moment. Finally, you can listen to our Threshold Meditation (see the link at the end of this chapter) to achieve a powerful threshold moment.

The Perineum Threshold

We can't talk about threshold moments without talking about *the* threshold moment in birth: the moment the baby stretches the perineum and pops out into the world—which is also the final threshold—mom and baby cross together. The perineum is that soft, delicate skin between the vagina and anus that must stretch for the baby's head and body to finally be born, so it is important to understand its energetics.

The perineum houses the first chakra (see Chapter 1). It holds the energy of survival, security, protection, and also fear. When the first chakra and perineum exude feelings of safety, trust, sovereignty, and courage, they are more likely to stretch effectively and beautifully during birth. However, if fear and stress are present in the first chakra, the energy of defensiveness manifests, which can cause physical tension in the perineum and restrict how much it can stretch. When these tissues can't sufficiently stretch in birth to allow for baby's body to push through, they tear or require episiotomy (a surgical cut by a doctor). You can think of this phenomenon as the energetic closing down of the fort to protect the treasure. Courage, on the other hand, offers deep stretch, opening, expansion, and vulnerability. Both scenarios are very normal and beautiful experiences of birth, but they show us on a physical level how our unconscious fears can restrict our physical birth experience. This is another reason why it is so important to face our fears before labor so we can have the most stretch and openness available to us.

Fear is a difficult gate that you may come up against time and time again in pregnancy and in labor. Using the tools and understandings in this chapter can help bring you more courage and sovereignty to the birthing space and give you a greater sense of empowerment down the path to motherhood.

Integration Practices

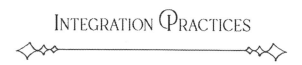

The following practices are intended to help you integrate the information of this chapter and apply it to your life now, so you can prepare to walk through this gate with courage and sovereignty when you're in labor. Take your time going through the practices that resonate the most with you and feel free to do them as often as you'd like.

Self-Love Activity: Create Courage Cards

For this activity, spend an afternoon with your inner Maiden. Reminisce about times you have felt courageous. What states arose within you? Did you feel brave? Strong? Empowered? Use this energy and allow it to fill your body before creating your courage cards.

This activity can be as crafty or as basic as you prefer. The purpose is to create at least 10 different index cards or postcards that cultivate the energy of courage and sovereignty within you. You can write words of encouragement, inspirational quotes, affirmations, jokes, meaningful stories, or make a collage or draw memories on each of the cards. Add anything else that puts your mind and body into a state of joy, courage, and determination. When complete, you can use them like playing cards or oracle cards during your labor to help walk you through this gate when you find that fear gets intense. Let these be gentle reminders to return to your power center in moments of fear.

INNER EXPLORATION JOURNAL PROMPTS

The following journal prompts are for you to explore and uncover the different challenges of this gate. The practice of journaling can be deeply healing and enlightening, so we encourage you to spend some time reading over the prompts to see which ones resonate with you. Look back at these often. You might notice that different journal prompts resonate at different times.

Fear

- What is the one thing I am most afraid of happening in labor from a physical perspective? From an emotional perspective? From a mental perspective? From a spiritual perspective?
- Where do these fears come from? Society? Family? Friends? Myself?
- What swords, a.k.a., coping mechanisms, have I used in the past to deal with/cope with /avoid/numb my fears? What would my life look like if I just suddenly threw all my swords out and faced my fears head on?
- What is the worst thing that could happen if I sacrificed my swords? What is the best thing that could happen? What is the most likely thing that could happen? Is this true? Am I seeing reality from the present moment, or am I living in the past/future?
- When I was growing up, what was the biggest fear my parents/caregiver had about parenthood or motherhood? Was this fear projected on me? If yes, how did that make me feel? Do I see these fears in myself? Do I project them onto others or onto my baby?
- How have my family's fears affected my own? Have my partner's fears affected my own?
- How did/do my parents deal with their fear? Do I deal with fear in the same way? Do I want to change this and raise my child differently? If so, how?
- Where in my life have I been trapped in the fear–pain cycle? What happened? How did I feel? How did I get out of it? If I could do it

differently, what would I do? Can I apply these lessons to labor? How can I remind myself of these lessons while I am in labor?

Sovereignty

- Do I speak up for myself and have agency in all aspects of my life? If not, where do I hand over my authority? To whom? Why do I do this?
- What emotion drives me to not have full sovereignty? How does fear play into this dynamic I have? Is this something I want to teach my child or transform for my child?
- What types of people do I have the most difficulty maintaining my sovereignty with- family members, partners, children, medical professionals, teachers, spiritual authority figures, police officers?
- What times in my life have I crossed this gate and been rewarded with a sense of courage and sovereignty? How did that feel? How did that affect my self-esteem?

GODDESS RITUAL: TRANSFORMING FEAR

This is a great ritual to do after considering or journaling the prompts above. In this ritual, all you need to do is spend some time with yourself. Find a quiet spot, somewhere you feel safe. This ritual is all about self-reflection and acknowledgment. It requires courage to face the things you are most afraid of.

What You Need:

- A few minutes of alone time
- A pen and paper if you want to journal during this ritual (although it's not necessary)

What to Do:

Spend a few minutes thinking about or journaling all your major fears. Focus in on one specific fear that worries you, especially in labor. Let the fear come into full expression as you hold that fear in your mind and walk through the following four steps.

1. **Recognize your fear** by experiencing it and naming it. You can say, "I am afraid of . . ." It's best to say this out loud if you can.
2. **Find where it lives** by asking yourself where this fear lives in your body. Where do you feel it physically? If you are having a hard time finding where it lives, ask yourself what parts of your body feel tense. Is your jaw clenched? Are your hands in fists? Looking for tense areas will give you clues as to where the fear lives for you. It might be in multiple areas.
3. **Witness your fear** by imagining it as a color, object, or symbol in your mind's eye. You can make it up or use the first thing that pops into your mind. Really take a look at it. What is it doing? Is it changing, moving, staying still? Just watch it without controlling it. Notice if other feelings come up and then witness those.
4. **Transform your fear** by spending a moment honoring this fear and asking what it is trying to protect. Tell your fear it is time for it to leave your body. Ask it if it needs to communicate anything else to you before it goes. When you feel ready, with your breath, imagine the fear loosening and releasing itself from its former home. For example, if your fear lives in your chest and you see it as barbed wire, imagine it being cut down and removed. Allow the pieces of your fear to be swept up into a pile of energy that no longer serves you. With one large exhale let that energy go.

This ritual can be done with all your fears, and you might have to do it multiple times for the same fear. Fear is tricky; the same fear can live in many places and look differently.

GODDESS RITUAL: MAIDEN-TO-MOTHER AFFIRMATION

Say the following affirmation as often as you like aloud, quietly or as a mantra over and over again as you transition from Maiden-to-Mother. Place your hands over your perineum or the base of spine and say: *"I am*

powerful and sovereign over all my fears and doubts. I face the unknown with
the courage of the billions of women who have birthed before me and will
birth after me."

THRESHOLD MEDITATION

In this meditation, you'll go on a short journey through the Gate of
Courage and Sovereignty to cross the threshold of transformation. This
is a perfect meditation if you are struggling to release and let go of fear.
The practice can be done after each journal prompt or daily until you feel
you have completed your transition. It is also a great meditation for labor
when those moments of fear show up. Visit www.laborlikeagoddess.com
to download it.

Final Thoughts

We are so proud of you for making it this far, Goddess, because this is
big, life-changing stuff and it takes a tremendous amount of courage just
to read through this first Gate of Transformation—so congratulations!
If you do nothing else, know that you've already moved through one
level of this journey. You are practically a professional! Well, okay, maybe
not, but doesn't it feel like it? We invite you to take your time doing the
Integration Practices and journal prompts that resonate with you. It's truly
a transformative process if you give yourself the time and space to explore
this gate. You deserve it!

~ CHAPTER III ~

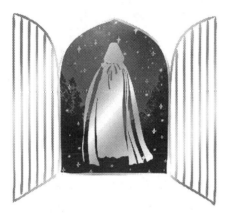

THE GATE
OF VULNERABILITY
FACING SHAME

It's tougher to be vulnerable than to actually be tough.

—*Rhianna*

The Maiden Goddess continued on the path to the Underworld for several more hours. With her newfound sense of courage, the noises of the night and dancing shadows no longer scared her. She welcomed them as entertainment as she journeyed. The night grew very cold, and it began to snow hard, and the Maiden tightened her cloak around her.

Before she knew it, she came upon another gate, much like the first one. Big, iron-clad, and enchanted. She knocked, and another old-woman Gatekeeper appeared, asking what business she had knocking on her gate. The Maiden answered, "I long to become a mother. I wish to go into the Underworld."

"Ah, yes, I see," said the Gatekeeper. "Then you must pass through this gate. And what will you give me in return for your passage? How about that beautiful, warm cloak you are wearing?"

"I can't give you my cloak," scoffed the Maiden. "That would be most inappropriate. I am naked underneath! I will be exposed, and everyone will see what I keep only for myself. How dare you ask for such a sacrifice? There must be something else."

The Gatekeeper only replied, "The cloak, Maiden. That is the sacrifice required. You will just have to learn to be naked and seen in your full truth and glory."

"This is not fair. I won't do it. Why are you treating me like this?" the Maiden Goddess cried, but the Gatekeeper said nothing.

Realizing that blaming the Gatekeeper wasn't going to help her, the Maiden took some time to wrestle with the idea of walking the rest of the way naked. She wasn't concerned with how the weather could affect her. No, she was much more concerned with the shame of it all. That level of vulnerability. But the Gatekeeper's words echoed in her mind, ". . . learn to be naked and seen in your full truth and glory."

Could she do that? It sounded really hard and awkward, but motherhood was all she wanted, so she agreed to the sacrifice. The Maiden Goddess removed her cloak, felt the icy chill on her skin, and the gates opened.

The shame she feared immediately fell over her, and she tried to cover her body with her hands. She contorted herself to cover up the parts she wished to remain hidden. But she knew she wouldn't be able to walk the rest of the way, avoiding her nudity. She was naked. That was a fact. And right then and there she decided to stop avoiding it and embrace it.

She said to herself, "I will not feel ashamed for my naked truth or the choices I make. I am a goddess, and I will be a mother. I'm going to walk through this gate with my head held high, to be seen by all, and to see by myself in all my glory."

And so she did. Naked, exposed, vulnerable, and without either her sword or her cloak, she crossed the threshold of this second gate— willingly, with courage and fierce vulnerability. She continued on her path, chin to the stars, and a smile on her lips. She eventually forgot that she was naked at all and found a new sense of inner strength she didn't realize she had."

The Symbol of the Cloak

On first read, the old Gatekeeper's request for the Maiden's cloak seems like a cruel sacrifice. It is snowing and cold, and the cloak is the only thing keeping her from freezing to death. Asking for it in exchange for passage is more like a death sentence than a fair trade, and this gate can definitely feel like that in labor. But the Gatekeeper knows something that not even the Maiden knows—the Maiden is much more capable than she realizes. The cloak was suppressing her, holding her back from her naked truth and blocking her from her true goddess power. The cloak would only hinder her and couldn't come on the journey to motherhood.

It is a terrifying prospect to lose her cloak and bare herself. The consequences of this sacrifice are threefold:

1. She loses a powerful boundary of protection between her own softness and the harsh reality of the world around her;
2. She loses her ability to cover her shame and hide from her truth; and
3. She is forced to stand in her own vulnerability, in full exposure.

And yet, she doesn't crumble under the weight of this sacrifice as she feared she might. No, the Maiden realizes the only way to walk through this gate is to *own* it all. Own everything about herself—her choices, her nakedness, her vulnerability—and walk through with pride and empowerment. What she feared would victimize her and make her suffer transforms into a powerful rallying cry of motherhood.

As women, we are asked to walk through the Gate of Vulnerability time and time again in pregnancy, labor, and motherhood. Sometimes, just like the Maiden, we find our courage and empowerment; we walk through this gate with our heads held high, and shame is transformed into a sense of pride. Other times, we resist the sacrifice and feel victimized by the exposure. Whenever victimization is present, emotional or psychological trauma tends to follow. The rest of this chapter describes the common habit or temptation of falling into victim mode when we are faced with vulnerability in our pregnancy and labor.

The Temptation to Feel Victimized

Whenever we go through an intense event or situation, it is our natural human instinct to look to blame someone else for our suffering. Little kids do it, adults do it, and politicians do it. It's as if we think that blaming someone else will ease our own suffering—and maybe it does for a moment, but we can't heal when we blame others. Because where there is blame, there is victimization. Whenever we blame someone (whether deserved or not), we avoid our own emotional responsibility, which undermines our sovereignty. And the detrimental consequence of doing this is that our pain and emotional and psychological sensitivity increase dramatically—something that can make any labor feel traumatic.

Birth is one of the most intense things we can go through in life and so blaming others while in the throes of contractions can be a very tempting coping mechanism (the metaphorical cloak), especially if we are in this habit of avoiding emotional responsibility. We've all heard the famous line from the movies, "You did this to me!" as a laboring woman screams at her husband. It's kinda funny as entertainment, but actually quite disempowering to the woman giving birth. By blaming her husband for something that she willingly agreed to, even if in a moment of anger or emotion, is actually one of the most deflating things she could do for herself in a moment where she needs the most inner power, encouragement, and oomph.

This kind of lashing out puts us in a "victim" mentality where we no longer have self-authority and are no longer at the helm of our birth experience—two very important components of an empowered birth experience. Birth is now something that is happening *to* us, rather than *with* us. Whenever we become victims to a situation, seeds of trauma can plant themselves into the experience and can cause problems for us as we step into motherhood.

We believe this is one of the reasons that 3,000 women a day experience some form of psychological trauma from their birth experience. It's not due to the physical marathon of labor, or the anticipation of a having baby, or even the loss of Maiden life, though all of those are big emotional and psychological transitions. No, the main source of trauma in birth comes from feeling victimized by the experience, rather than empowered by it—no matter what has actually occurred in the timeline of events.

As doulas, we've witnessed every single kind of birth imaginable—hospital, emergency, breech, in taxi cabs and cars, at home and in birth centers, toilet births—you name it. We've also seen trauma affect all kinds of moms, no matter what the situation or birthing preference. The one thing that has been true for those affected with trauma is a sense of feeling victimized by the experience, rather than invigorated. It's become very clear to us that avoiding or minimizing psychological birth trauma has nothing to do with *where, how* or *with whom* we birth, and everything to do with how much we've *owned* our experience, emotions, and inner reality. It really comes down to what is happening in our minds and belief systems.

So, as you move through this gate even now in pregnancy, it is important to start noticing your own thoughts, habits, and patterns that tempt you into victim mode, so you can heal and step into an empowered attitude when this gate appears in labor.

Small Ways We Unknowingly Victimize Ourselves

It's human nature to victimize ourselves now and then, without realizing what we are doing. Sometimes it is referred to as self-sabotage, negative thinking, or a bad attitude. In labor, we refer to it as "falling into a victim mode." Whenever we avoid our own truth or expressing it to the world, we are actually creating a low-level victim mentality, albeit unconsciously or out of habit, whenever we want to protect ourselves from others or feel helpless, misunderstood, or shamed.

Essentially, this is what the Maiden Goddess was doing by hiding underneath her cloak, protecting herself from being seen in her full glory. She is a goddess and doesn't live in a world where modesty is a social construct, so why cover up? Perhaps because she had the same fears that many of us battle: of being "too much," "too big," "too bright," "too powerful."

Or perhaps she wished to avoid the exposure, vulnerability and possible shame she would feel if others couldn't "handle her," so she chose to dress down, cover up, and hide to avoid conflict or discomfort.

As women, we often do the same, especially in labor, when we feel vulnerable. We fall into the habit of dimming our light or watering down our expressions to avoid uncomfortable feelings, conflict, or inner shames to "just get through it". As doulas, we've seen many women bite their tongue or agree to a procedure just to avoid the conflict or the fear of rejection. This may have been a successful coping mechanism in maidenhood, but this attitude has no place in motherhood. As mothers, we can't afford to fall into victim-mode as we need to be fierce and sovereign caretakers of our babies. The Gatekeeper understood that the only way for the Maiden Goddess to break past this conditioning was to face herself and her naked truth, and we must do the same to walk through this gate.

In pregnancy, we have many opportunities to cross this gate over and over again. Pregnancy can often feel like one big Gate of Vulnerability.

Our bodies change so much that our metaphorical cloaks containing our old ways of staying small can no longer contain our expansion. Our bellies and feet swell, we get bigger, thicker, wider. It is almost physically impossible to hide our full pregnant glory behind clothes or try to make ourselves small. It just ain't happening. So, we have the choice to own it and walk through the gate or to resist it and risk being traumatized by the experience of expansion.

It is easier for some to walk through this gate and incredibly difficult for others. It all depends upon how we deal with our own truth, our own feelings of shame, our own vulnerability and whether we allow ourselves to be seen as complete women (the good, the bad, and the ugly). The journal prompts at the end of this chapter will help you discover your own relationship with victimization and vulnerability. But before we get there, let's talk about shame.

The Shame Game

To remove our metaphorical cloaks, the things that keep us from being in our full light, we have to allow ourselves to be vulnerable. However, shame is one of the biggest barriers to vulnerability and one of the biggest reasons for slipping into victim mode. Wherever there is birth trauma, we find shame as the culprit. So, understanding what shame is, where it comes from, and how to work with it can make or break having an empowered labor. Women who get friendly with their shame and own it have the most fulfilling labor and delivery experiences, which is why we believe it is so important to deal with shame in pregnancy while we have the emotional resources to dig deep and heal.

The best way to understand shame is to see all the places and times shame bombards our psyche—which, as women, is often. We get shame from everything and everywhere—social norm understandings, entertainment, advertisements, religion, family, parenting, and even from ourselves. That's because, as humans, we love to use shame as a tool of punishment to police each other. It's like an invisible switch we use to whack those who step out of line, go against the status quo, or break the social rules —including ourselves. We've got laws for civil structure and shame for social structure. And it's a brilliant tool that has served us well for millennia. But, as you can imagine, when used inappropriately or abusively, it causes deep striations of pain, blows to self-worth, and psychological trauma. The reason for this is down to the mechanics of shame—which is one part psychological influence and one part emotional reaction. The psychological part starts with the person doing the shaming. The person seeking to control a behavior by undermining another's sense of self-worth, adequacy in the group dynamic or honor, whether intentional or not. The emotional part completes the dynamic with the one receiving the shaming: the one experiencing a painful feeling of humiliation or distress caused by the self-consciousness of wrong or foolish behavior. This doesn't have to be cruel or abusive. We do it all the time as parents.

For example, let's say the social norm is that little girls should behave like little ladies and keep their dresses down. At home, Sally, who is three, is allowed to run and be as she pleases. When her parents have friends over, and Sally lifts up her dress like she always does at home, her mother scolds her and says, "Put your dress down, Sally; why would you do that? That's not very ladylike." Sally is confused, and feels shame, but doesn't understand why. In this example, the mother is seeking to control her child's behavior around guests to obey social norms. She undermines Sally's self-worth with her question, "Why would you do that?" even though she knows that Sally does it all the time, and that she allows it. That is the psychological component of shame, the first part. Sally is confused and feels that she has done something wrong but isn't quite sure why and, the second part—the emotional reaction—settles in. Sally concludes in her young mind that it's not okay to be herself around people outside of the family.

Shame is so interesting because it is one of the few emotions that requires the interaction of two people to ignite. It takes two to tango. All our other emotions naturally arise and don't require outside instigation. For example, from the time we are newborns, we can experience fear, joy, happiness, anxiety, and so on, without any other interaction. Shame requires an external force—a psychological starter.

So, as we explore and face shame, it is important to know that it doesn't originate within us but begins with someone else putting that shame on us. The greatest lie shame tells us is that we aren't good enough, and humans are simply not born with this instinct. Rather, society, family, parents, teachers, religious authorities, entertainment, and friends put that notion in our heads. Shame isn't natural, yet we all subscribe to it because it binds us together socially.

This example with Sally is a very simple way of illustrating how a small interaction of shame can affect our sense of value and worth. But shame can also take a dark turn and be incredibly abusive and traumatic. Traumatic shame can become so indoctrinated in how we view ourselves that we actually believe we are inherently wrong, broken, or faulty. We start to experience severe self-worth and self-esteem issues, and the trauma of this painful shame affects nearly every aspect of our lives, including birth and motherhood. If you think you may have traumatic shame, we highly recommend working with a trained professional counselor, therapist, or healer to help you face those belief systems. This can be one of the most empowering things you can do to support yourself, your labor, and your baby (see the Resources).

But trauma aside, shame, in general, affects our vulnerability. If we handled shame well as children and were able to naturally own our own flaws and truths, vulnerability would be much easier to access as adults. However, if shame was difficult to face as children, and we ran away from it, hid from it, avoided it, lied to ourselves about it or punished ourselves for it, then we are probably doing the same thing now as adults. It's this pattern that can cause some upset during labor.

A DOULA'S BIRTH STORY

Sarah was a new mom and excited about bringing her baby into the world. She was deeply religious and conservative, and she trusted wholeheartedly in God's will. She attended birth classes, hired me as her doula, and prepared for the physical aspects of labor. But when we talked about nudity or the primal nature of birth, she always blushed and said, "That won't be a problem for me." A few weeks later, she called me after laboring all night and wanted me to come over as things were picking up. When I arrived, her husband answered the door and looked worried. Sarah had locked herself in her room and wouldn't let him in. I went upstairs and knocked, and could hear her sobbing and hyperventilating on the other side. She was in a full panic attack. She opened the door for me and told me how excruciating her contractions were. I could see the terror in her eyes. She was scared. We spent the next 40 minutes, focusing on breathing to calm her down and get back into the rhythm.

When she felt a little better, she confided in me that her husband heard her "moan like a beast," and she was mortified. She locked herself in her room and waited for me to come. When asked about her pain level before the moan, she said she was doing really great—she was actually enjoying riding the waves—but then she made "that sound" and everything got intense and hard. After some listening, I said, "If you made a noise like that to birth your baby, it must be holy because God is looking over this birth." At that moment, a sense of relief came over her, and her perspective changed. She reframed her "shameful noise" into a prideful holy sound in her mind. A deep sense of self-acceptance came into the space. For the rest of her labor, she moaned and howled, without feeling self-conscious, and her baby was born gently and with so much love. Sarah recalls the only "really painful" part of her birth was when she locked herself in her room when she refused to face her own shame.

As witnessed by Alexandria Moran

Nudity, Shame, and the Garden of Eden

Now that we understand how shame works in our society, let's start to unpack how shame has been taught to us from religion. The Abrahamic religions—Christianity, Judaism, and Islam—all start with the same origin story; the story of the Garden of Eden.

In this story, Adam and Eve roam the garden of paradise, naked and unaware of their own shame. They are told specifically not to eat from the Tree of Knowledge. But Eve, tempted by a snake, takes an apple and eats it against God's will, and then gives it to Adam to eat. Upon discovering this, God punishes Adam and Eve. They are cast out of the garden of paradise. Shame falls upon them, they immediately experience their own nudity, and Eve is punished with pain in childbirth. Adam and Eve leave the garden and begin to procreate our humanity.

Wow. This story hits like a ton of bricks when we look at its symbolism and consequences as it relates to birth. The connection between shame and nudity began the moment that Eve, a woman, disobeys the authority figure, God. *Exile* and *shame* became the tools of punishment for the crime of disobedience. We see this dynamic play out even now in our modern-day society, where women are afraid of being "too much" or wanting too much, like Eve, and being outcast for it. We also see where shame is used as a punishment for disobeying societal rules or authority figures.

A DOULA'S BIRTH STORY

As a doula, I've held the space for many women as they bravely stood up to their doctors when they felt like they were being bullied for their alternative birth choices. I've even advocated for many of them, with conviction, compassion, and strength. I had always assumed that I would have that same ferocity when it was my time to be a mom-to-be. But as I grew bigger and bigger in pregnancy, I felt more and more vulnerable.

I found myself feeling intense shame when questioned about my choices and being extremely meek in the presence of my doctors. It surprised me how my own old and emotional wounding around shame and authority showed up so strongly.

At one appointment, I had insisted on waiting for a particular test and then somehow ended up agreeing to it—even when everything in my body was screaming "No!"

I walked out of the doctor's appointment in tears and couldn't believe that I, of all people, felt victimized. I felt a deep sense of shame and self-betrayal, and I couldn't understand how I could be so fierce for others and a doormat when it came to fighting for my own welfare. I then realized how this gate was showing up for me, and I committed to doing the inner work to heal my fears and shames around authority and sovereignty with my medical team.

At my next appointment, I stood my ground and still felt unheard. I decided to part ways with my care-provider and did so from a place of empowerment. As soon as I stopped abandoning myself and faced my inner shame, I took back my sovereignty and self-respect.

As experienced by Alexandria Moran

But there is something else that may not be as obvious that is revealed in the Garden of Eden story: harboring shame can cause pain in childbirth. As doulas, we have seen this phenomenon firsthand and know this secret: the more shame we experience while in labor, the more pain we feel with each contraction. Conversely, the more open vulnerability we allow ourselves to feel in labor, the more pleasure and empowerment we experience with each contraction. But God gave Eve an out: she could choose to not fall victim to the shame that was cast upon her, but rather face it, own it and integrate it to continue to experience fulfilling pain-free births. The Maiden in our story discovered how to do this and held her head high as she walked through the Gate of Vulnerability—and we can too.

Shame and Birth

We can't seem to escape how shame and birth go hand in hand because shame sets up shop in the womb and the second chakra—just as fear lives in the perineum and the first chakra (see Chapter 1). Birth is nothing if not a full-womb experience. We are stretching, pushing, contracting, and expanding all the organs, ligaments, and bones of the pelvis while simultaneously activating all the energy, memories and traumas of shame that is held in those organs, ligaments, and bones. So, needless to say, feelings of shame show up in every single laboring experience, whether we try to repress it or not. Even mothers who have fully anesthetized C-sections still experience an opportunity to face their own shame in recovery as those physical and energetic parts heal. No matter how hard we try, we can't separate the two.

The only thing we can do is control how we react to the shame that shows up. As we've described, shame exists on a sliding scale of emotion from simple embarrassment to full-fledged trauma. In birth, it can show up on one side of the spectrum—let's say embarrassment from farting in front of a nurse (which seems like a small shame) —to the higher end of the spectrum, let's say sexual trauma triggered from a cervical check (which seems like an intense shame). The level of shame isn't what determines the pain level of the laboring mother. It's actually how she reacts to the shame that determines whether she experiences more or less pain.

So, a mother who experiences severe humiliation from a social faux pas, like a fart, will experience more pain than a mother who is only slightly affected by the trigger of sexual trauma. The difference between the two experiences is determined by how comfortable we are with our own feelings of shame, no matter where they fall on the spectrum.

This is a big reason why the Gatekeeper urges the Maiden Goddess to face her shame and get comfortable with her own inner truth. It is only when we make friends with our own feelings of shame, and maybe even sympathize with them, that we can avoid unnecessary pain in childbirth. When we resist our shame, we abandon our truth, keep ourselves small, and constrict the blood flow to the womb. This makes it much harder to ride the waves of contractions and the waves of shame that show up in birth.

A DOULA'S BIRTH STORY

Brianna was so excited about becoming a new mom, and she had prepared herself for the mental and emotional fear of the pain of childbirth as well as how her life would look as a mother. The one thing Brianna didn't think to prepare for was the shame that can arise during labor. Brianna was a very modest woman and described herself as "a prude and wholesome." After talking with her during our postpartum visit, I asked her what the hardest obstacle she had to face during her labor was. Her answer surprised me: "Being semi-nude in front of my husband, myself, and the medical staff." She told me that in the first moment of her labor when she was starting to feel the need to get naked, she felt scared and ashamed to show her body. What would her husband think, showing off her body to strangers? By the time transition was happening, she said she no longer cared. She felt this urge for a reason, and she went with it. At that moment, she knew that being ashamed of her naked body was holding her back from experiencing her birth fully.

As witnessed by Lauren Mahana

Shame and Judgment

As we can surmise from the Garden of Eden, shame can't exist without judgment. God cast his judgment onto Adam and Eve, and shame was the punishment. The two feed each other, and they are always connected. We often hold back from publicly shaming other people, but we don't have a problem secretly judging them. Since shame and judgment go hand in hand, when we judge others, we shame ourselves. Read that again.

It's a way of self-policing by drawing a comparison with others. It's kinda brilliant. Let's take the example of a man who is very overweight, taking a lot of time in the checkout line. We might not shame him, by saying out loud, "Hurry up, you fat slob!" No, we are too nice for that. But we may secretly judge him in our minds—surveying his girth, his hygiene, his heavy breathing, his slow walking. We may pass judgment about his character based on his physical appearance, and we do it on autopilot, whether we admit it to ourselves or not. Our judgment seems like it's about *him*, but really, it's our own judgment about how we feel about our own bodies, and by judging him, we are sort of self-policing to keep ourselves from ever getting *that big*, holding up checkout lines, and inconveniencing others (what we deem shameful behavior). Our judgment of someone else feeds the shame we have about ourselves and our ideas of the world.

This happens all the time in mommy circles too, where women judge each other as an emotional salve to avoid feeling their own inadequacies and shame around motherhood. But what if we instead just got real and faced our own feelings of shame? Owned our insecurities and embraced the truth of who we are? We bet that many more mommies would feel better and more supported by their tribe. There would be a deeper level of emotional intimacy between the mommies because it would feel more like a safe space to gather.

If you are reading all of this and just can't seem to find where you hide from yourself or what shame you carry, we invite you to start to look at where you judge other people or yourself. Judgment is a metaphorical cloak—just a way to avoid facing our own shames—and it is a great string to tug on to discover our deeper truths. We can't cross this threshold of vulnerability like a goddess if we keep getting caught in the judgment-shame cycle. Later in this chapter, you'll find some Integration Practices and journal prompts to help you crawl out of this unhealthy habit.

I'm a Bad Mother—the #1 Shame

Whether we admit it or not, the number-one shame we generally have as mothers is being seen or seeing ourselves as a *bad mother.* This shame usually kicks in during pregnancy as we make decisions about *what kind of* birth we will have, *where* we will birth, *what* procedures we accept, *if* we go back to work, how soon, will we breastfeed, etc. Fear of failing at motherhood can be overwhelming, and the shame of holding the "bad mother" title can be life-limiting for any woman.

It seems like every choice we make as a mother is tinged with shame or judgment, no matter what we choose. The only way to win at this endless game of shame and judgment is to face it head-on and own it. Allowing our choices to speak for themselves, and finding a sense of pride in so doing is one of the most powerful things we can do as mothers, and it teaches our children that they don't have to play the shame game either.

Shame and Vulnerability

Nevertheless, shame can be so difficult to deal with because it requires a level of vulnerability that we are just not taught how to embrace. This is because shame usually begins in our psyche when we are young, when we're at our most impressionable and vulnerable. Because of this, we have to choose to return to that state, at least emotionally, to shift that shame into pride. As we see in the Maiden Goddess story, she must become vulnerable first by removing her cloak and exposing herself before she can even look at her shame, let alone transform it and walk over the threshold as a new and empowered person.

Vulnerability is always the first step in facing our shame. It requires us to look at our truths, the sources of the shame, the truth of why we continue to shame ourselves, the truth of how we avoid our shame or hide from it, and the truth of how we lie to ourselves about it. Vulnerability creates the openness necessary to release ourselves from these shackles of shame, so we can lift our chins high and transform ourselves.

If we are too hardened through years of shaming, trauma, low self-esteem, and poor support, being vulnerable can seem like an almost impossible task. It is the biggest sacrifice, the biggest ask, the biggest risk. If this resonates with you, we highly recommend that you seek some professional and compassionate support to help you face your shame (See Recommended Resources). Professional support can be a powerful way to feel safe enough to reach the level of vulnerability required to take an honest look at your shame. We promise that by doing so, by getting comfortable with your own shame stories, you will not only empower your birth experience, but will also make pain management much easier. Trust us. We've seen even the most emotionally protective and hardened women find the courage and vulnerability to transform shame into pride. We believe you can too.

How to Walk Through the Gate of Vulnerability

We can't talk about shame, vulnerability, victimization, and judgment without talking about boundaries. These are the invisible borders between what's our "stuff" (i.e., responsibilities, emotions, thoughts, beliefs, needs) and another's. The integrity, strength, and clarity of our boundaries teach others how they can treat us and what is appropriate when interacting with us. When we have good, strong boundaries, we find that people tend to respect and honor our decisions more because they can clearly understand where the boundary is between them and us. When our boundaries are unclear or non-existent, we find that people tend to take advantage of us more often, and it can be difficult to speak up or feel important. So, learning how to create good boundaries is an important step in emotional maturity and a necessary aspect to face shame with a sense of empowerment, rather than victimization.

When we first learn how to establish emotional boundaries, especially if we have a history of letting others walk all over us, we are like a swinging pendulum. We start off on one side, where we may be really bad at creating any boundaries whatsoever, and then swing to the other side where our boundaries are the envy of Fort Knox. We don't let anyone or anything in. When we are first learning how to be vulnerable, it feels safer to make these Fort-Knox type of boundaries that are strong and rigid. It's a great first start as we dip our toes into the pool of the vulnerability. But just like the Maiden Goddess, we can't wade in the shallow waters if we want to become conscious and embodied mothers. We must completely submerge ourselves in empowered vulnerability. That means learning how to make healthy boundaries.

Healthy boundaries are both strong and flexible, just like the branches of a tree. They can bend, they can sway, they can move and change. They are neither rigid nor loose. This is because healthy boundaries, by nature, should change moment to moment. What is right at one moment, may feel off or wrong a moment later. So, our boundaries should be adaptable enough to move with us in life. If they are too rigid, we may be saying "NO" out of habit, or fear, and missing out on things that could be helpful or fulfilling. If our boundaries are too loose and formless, like a scarf blowing in the wind, they can't hold our no's and so we can't be in our truth moment to moment, either. We have to find a firm but flexible middle ground.

Learning to relax our boundaries and still stay authentic and true in the moment is a skill that requires practice. It is usually not something we can grasp overnight because it takes some trial and error. But as with any adventure, we have to be willing to put ourselves out there to fail, mess up, be too loose with our boundaries, and be too rigid until we find the perfect Goldilocks groove to move and shift with us through life.

A DOULA'S BIRTH STORY

This is a personal story from my first birth. Right after I was admitted to the hospital, I was told I needed an IV. I wasn't thrilled, but my water had broken early into my labor, and I was becoming dehydrated. When the nurse came in to put in the line, she was friendly, a little sarcastic, but overall quite pleasant. While she was getting her things together, I mentioned that I have very deep veins, and the one in my arm was really hard to get.

The second I told her this, it was like flipping a switch. Her attitude toward me completely shifted. She began to lecture me on finding veins and that she would be able to find it—that I had no clue about placing an IV. While she was telling me this, I began to feel ashamed for saying anything. The nurse was making me feel like I didn't know my own body. While this was all swirling around in my head, the nurse attempted to find my vein three times. After the fourth try, she gave up and placed the IV into my hand. My arm was already bruising, and I was starting to feel pain before my contractions had even begun. She was still talking about how she was great at placing IVs and how silly I was for planning an unmedicated birth. At this point, I was barely listening to her, because I had come to a major realization: that I was the only one who could make me feel this way. She was just projecting her own insecurities onto me, and I didn't have to stand for it. Mid-sentence, I asked the nurse to please leave because I needed to be alone.

While she was heading to the door, she made another snide comment of unwanted advice, and right at that moment I asked her not to come back and that she would not be in my birthing space. (I might have said this in a less friendly way, I can't remember my exact words.) She looked backed stunned but respected my wishes, and that was it. I had formed my first boundary for my sacred birthing space. Creating that boundary was the first of many and it allowed me to feel empowered throughout my labor and delivery.

Experienced by Lauren Mahana

Having strong, yet flexible boundaries in each and every moment makes vulnerability so much easier to cultivate, and it's pretty hard to be victimized when our boundaries are true and responsive. Just like Lauren's story, learning to establish boundaries at the moment a boundary is crossed is true mastery of the Maiden-self and a beautiful way to cross the Gate of Vulnerability. This gate asks you to be vulnerable enough to face your own inner truths, including shame. But to even see your shame, you must choose to become vulnerable and open enough to see it before it can be faced and integrated.

Each time you embrace vulnerability, truths and shames will show up, and you have a choice: to cower, hide, resist, ignore, avoid, and push back OR to embrace, encourage, lean in, face straight on, and fully own the experience. You get to choose what you will do. Will you be a victim or a victor? A seeker or a hider? Will you be weakened or strengthened? Will you be discouraged or empowered? That's what is so cool about each of these gates . . . the power is always in your hands.

So, walking through the Gate of Vulnerability, you're being asked to face things that keep you from being vulnerable—shame, judgment, and victimization. You're being asked to allow vulnerability to soften and open your boundaries so you can experience the reward of inner strength and acceptance. The Integration Practices at the end of this chapter are very helpful ways of breaking down rigid barriers to vulnerability safely and healthily. We highly recommend trying them out. If you are ready to start to explore your current feelings around shame, victimization, and judgment, now, while you have the emotional resources and energy, we have put together a list of journal prompts to help facilitate your journey. These are questions that have created great emotional breakthroughs for our clients and for ourselves.

Tuning into your womb space is another great way to emotionally and energetically embrace the power and transform the pain in this gate. Doing womb healing, hip circles, belly dancing, and talking to your womb are all great ways to connect with your vulnerability and give any shame you're holding a chance to express itself in a safe environment, rather than having it come screaming out during labor. It is also a great way to give your baby a healing too since he or she is steeped in the fluids of the womb. And in healing the womb of shame, our children are less likely to suffer from the same stories.

Finally, creating healthy boundaries is the best way of transforming any shame into a source of personal power. In our story, the Maiden Goddess does an amazing job of setting a boundary with her own thoughts. She acknowledges her shame, even placates it for a moment, and then realizes that it is unhelpful. So, she sets a boundary and says to herself, "No, I will not feel ashamed for my naked truth nor the choices I make. I am a goddess, and I will be a mother. I'm going to walk through this gate with my head held high, in all my glory." This one moment of setting a strong-yet-flexible boundary is the exact thing she needs to cross over the threshold. She says *no* to the lies that shame wants to tell her, and she rewrites the thoughts she wants to have! If you can learn to do this daily before labor begins, you will walk through the Gate of Vulnerability with ease when it matters the most.

Integration Practices

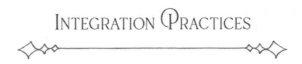

The following practices are intended to help you integrate the information of this chapter and apply it to your life now, so you can walk through this gate with pride and have strong, healthy boundaries while in labor. Take your time going through the practices that resonate the most with you and feel free to do them as often as you'd like.

Self-Love Activity: Mirror Gazing

When you are alone, stand naked in front of a mirror. Examine yourself as neutrally as possible. If judgment shows up, write it down, and get it out of your head. Then, return to gazing on your body. Circle your hips, move, watch your body shift, and change with your movement. Notice what is beautiful about your body. Notice what you love about your body. Notice what you have maybe neglected and could love more.

Next, stand straight and stare at your own eyes. Blink as much as you need to but don't break your gaze. Try to stay eye-locked with yourself for three minutes straight. Set a timer, so you don't have to break your gaze to look at the time. Notice what feelings come up for you as you stare into your own eyes. What vulnerabilities show up? What insecurities? You don't have to figure them out, just notice and keep gazing. At the end of the three minutes, journal everything that comes up for you.

Self-Love Activity: Eye-Gazing With a Partner

Now you are going to eye-gaze with another person. You can start with your clothes on. Stand in front of a trusted friend or partner about 12 inches apart. Don't touch, but lock gazes. Set a timer for three minutes. This can feel very awkward at first, but keep staring. Don't break eye contact. Allow any uncomfortable energies to melt away as you both stare into each other's eyes. Notice what feelings come up. Try not to talk, just stare and notice. At the end of the three minutes, spend some time journaling what comes up for you. After you've journaled, share your feelings with your partner. What was comfortable, what wasn't, what felt awkward, what felt good. Then hold space for your partner to share with you. To up the intensity of this exercise, eye-gaze with your lover naked. This unveils a whole new level of vulnerability.

INNER EXPLORATION JOURNAL PROMPTS

The following journal prompts are for you to explore and uncover the different challenges of this gate. The practice of journaling can be deeply healing and enlightening, so we encourage you to spend some time reading over the prompts to see which ones resonate with you. Look back at these often. You might notice that different journal prompts resonate at different times.

Victimization

- Have I ever blamed someone else when I felt out of control? If yes, how did that make me feel?
- Have I ever been blamed for someone else's emotions? If so, how did/does that make me feel?
- Do I take responsibility for my own emotions? If not, in what circumstances do I not take responsibility?
- Do I ever feel like I have to do everything on my own?
- Am I victimized by a lack of support around me?
- Have I ever felt victimized before? If so, what happened? How did this experience make me feel? Was I able to transform it into empowerment?
- Have I ever been a victim of a crime, abuse, or neglect? If so, how has that affected the way I feel about myself? How has it affected my vulnerability?
- When was a time that I felt victimized, but I was able to transform it into empowerment? What happened? How did that make me feel?
- When was a time that I felt victimized, and it turned into a trauma that I still haven't overcome? What happened? What is keeping me from transforming this experience into one that is helpful for me?

Shame

- What am I ashamed of? In my body? In my personality? In my mental acuity? In my social skills? In my mothering?
- What am I proud of? In my body? In my personality? In my mental acuity? In my social skills? In my mothering?
- What are my personal metaphorical "cloaks" that keep me from seeing my own truth and basking in my glory?
- Why am I afraid of facing my truth and my shame?
- The lie my shame tells me is: [_fill in your answer_].
- The biggest shame I want to avoid in birth is: [_fill in your answer_].
- I would just die if my partner/husband/family/doctor found out: [_fill in your answer_] about me.
- The places I still play small in my life are: [_fill in your answer_].
- Do I feel like I have to control myself through self-shaming? Where does this come from? Who else in my life does this?
- When was the first time I remember being shamed? What happened? Who shamed me? How did it make me feel? Does it still affect my life?
- Who was the first person I shamed? What happened? Who shamed me? How did it make me feel? Does it still affect my life?

Judgment

- What are the last five things I judged about myself?
- What are the last five things I judged in others?
- Do any of these judgments connect to my own insecurities and shames?
- Is there a better way to self-police than through judgment? Who judged me growing up? What did they say? How did it feel? Do I believe their assessment of me? How do these judgments affect my own self-esteem?

Goddess Ritual: Sacral Healing and Womb Connection

This ritual isn't just about letting go of what has wounded your womb, but how to integrate those experiences into your body. By allowing these wounds to become self-healing tools, you will help honor every experience you have had as a part of who you are today.

What You Need:

- A pen and two sheets of paper
- A candle and a lighter or matches
- A nonflammable bowl

What to Do:

On your piece of paper, draw or write how you feel about your womb. Put down the first things that come to your mind. Do these feelings emit a strong sense of self-love or not? Really look at it and see the true essences of your depiction.

On the other piece of paper, draw or write how you want to feel about your womb. Now compare the two. What are the differences? How can you create a connection of love to your womb space? Meditate on this. Close your eyes and imagine how you can repair your womb.

Light your candle or take a match or lighter and burn the paper with your first depiction of your womb. While it burns honor what it has given you. Honor the idea that your womb needs to be loved and cared for.

Allow the paper to burn to ashes in a bowl. When the embers have died out, take your ashes and plant them into Mother Earth (outside in your yard, the woods, a park, or in a house plant). Allow the soil to transmute the energy into the love your womb and all wombs deserve to have.

Goddess Ritual: Maiden-to-Mother Affirmation

Say the following affirmation as often as you like aloud, quietly, or as a mantra over and over again as you transition from Maiden-to-Mother.

Place your hands over your womb and say: *"I am strong and divinely powerful when I allow myself to soften into vulnerability!"*

THRESHOLD MEDITATION

In this meditation, you'll go on a short journey through the Gate of Vulnerability to face shame, judgment, and victimization. This is a perfect meditation if you are struggling to let go of shame. This practice can be done after each journal prompt or daily until you feel complete in your transition. It is also a great meditation to put on during labor when those moments of shame show up. Visit www.laborlikeagoddess.com to download it.

Final Thoughts

We are so proud of you for making it through this chapter. We touched on some heavy topics and hopefully woke within you a desire to explore your emotional Underworld a little deeper to best prepare yourself for the most fulfilling birth experience. We also hope that when shame shows up in birth, as it always does, you will be equipped with the tools to witness and process it in the moment. We encourage you to explore the Integration Practices to help you do the necessary, courageous, and empowering work to strip naked and own the glory of your own truth, just like the Maiden Goddess. We see you, woman! Shine that bright light and release all shame!

CHAPTER IV

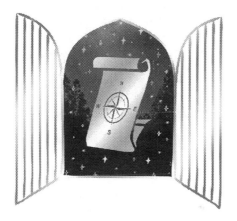

THE GATE
OF EXPECTATIONS
RELEASING CONTROL

Sometimes you have to let go of the picture of what you thought life would be like and learn to find joy in the story you are actually living.

—*Rachel Marie Martin, The Brave Art of Motherhood*

The Maiden Goddess walked for hours with her head held high, naked and without her sword. She felt confident in her path because her mother had given her a map of the Underworld. Everywhere she looked, it was just darkness and disorientation, so referring to the map kept her mind away from the fears and shames that could have crept in. She was so focused on the map that she nearly walked right into the next gate.

This gate was just like the previous two and so the Maiden Goddess knocked, apprehensive about what sacrifice she would need to make this time. Another wise, old Gatekeeper appeared asking her what business she had knocking on her door at this hour of the night.

"I long to become a mother. I wish to go to the Underworld. Please let me pass," the Maiden Goddess said.

The Gatekeeper surveyed this naked woman and noticed her hand quivering from the cold with a map in its grasp.

"Ah, yes, I see," said the Gatekeeper. "Then you will need to walk through this gate. I will let you pass. But only if you give me that map you have in your hand."

"Oh no, I'm sorry I can't give you this map. I need it to get to the Underworld. To become a mother. It's why I'm on this journey. This is the only way I can get there, and I can't afford to get lost. No. Anything else, it's yours."

The Gatekeeper's eyes widened at the Maiden Goddess' desperation and only replied, "The map, Maiden. That is the sacrifice required. You will just have to learn to find your way from within."

"What kind of riddle is this?!" the Maiden Goddess asked herself. Aimlessly walking to the Underworld without a sword and cloak wasn't *what she had signed up for. She was beginning to feel that this was too much sacrifice.*

She stomped her feet and had a few moments of anger, despair, frustration, and hopelessness. How was she expected to get anywhere in this darkness without a map? But then, she heard the calling within her womb to be brave and to learn to trust, and at that moment, she knew she could give up her expectations and find a new way.

"Okay," the Maiden Goddess said as she handed over the map. The Gatekeeper looked pleased by her willingness, and she opened the gate. As the Maiden Goddess passed over the threshold, she said to herself, "I trust my heart to find my way, because this calling to become a mother is a Divine one. I release how I thought this journey would go and embrace it as it is."

And with this newfound sense of trust, the Maiden Goddess continued on her journey into the Underworld.

The Map

When we prepare for anything in life, and especially for labor and birth, we want a map to help us get to our final destination. After all, just imagine trying to get anywhere without Google—we'd end up aimlessly wandering around, lost. Maps are important when we are on a journey, so why then does the Maiden Goddess have to give up hers?

Well, what the Maiden Goddess doesn't realize just yet is that she has already reached her destination: she's on the journey to the Underworld. In her mind, the destination is *becoming a mother,* but the Gatekeeper wisely knows that the journey *is* the destination, so, a map is neither needed nor useful. In fact, just like the sword and the cloak, the map has become an obsolete tool that she clings to unnecessarily. The Gatekeeper knows that the map may actually hinder her ability to navigate because the journey is an internal one.

The same can be said about women in labor. Despite the current trend of birth plans, once we arrive at our births—meaning labor has started—no birth plan can help us navigate what shows up, because it is unknown. Labor is completely out of our control. It is in the hands of our babies and the Divine. The only control we truly have in birth is how we move through the Gates of Transformation, how we react to the surprises that arise, and how easily we release our expectations. The Gatekeeper teaches us that clinging to a map, even a carefully crafted birth plan, can actually keep us from tuning into our own intuition and successfully navigating the ebbs and flows of labor.

By sacrificing her map, the Maiden Goddess must *trust* herself and birth AND learn how to navigate without external guidance. When she hands over the map, she is forced to look within to problem-solve, face unknown challenges, trust her instincts, and trust her intuition over some pre-destined outcome. Without someone else's directions, she is free to create her own map as dictated by her own experiences. In birth, this can feel like an incredibly scary and impossible scenario if we are so attached to a plan that we don't have faith in our inner ability to feel, sense, and flow with labor. As we move through the Gates of Transformation, each sacrifice asks us to rely more deeply on ourselves, rather than on outside tools to birth our babies. And, as doulas, we know that the biggest tool that gets moms stuck in the gates is their attachment to their birth plans and birth expectations.

Birth Plans and Expectations

Most childbirth preparation courses promote birth plans as a way to ensure empowered labor and to start the process of self-advocacy in pregnancy. From a logical perspective, birth plans make a lot of sense; they provide a set of rules, a structure, and written desires for *how* we want birth to unfold. Birth plans can give us a sense of control when planning our intentions and communicating our wants and needs to medical personnel or other people on the birth team. From this perspective, birth plans are amazing and incredibly helpful!

When used for their original purpose—to provide a loose framework for our intention for birth—birth plans are a positive tool. However, a lot of times, birth plans can warp into the be-all and end-all of how we expect birth to go, and that is when we can get ourselves in trouble. We can do this either consciously or subconsciously. We've had many clients, like our story about Debbie below, who very consciously attach themselves to their birth plans. But many moms do so unconsciously, and that's when surprise in labor can feel crushing and out of nowhere.

When we start to attach rigid expectations to childbirth, we move out of the space of using a birth plan as a helpful tool and begin to use it as a harmful psychological crutch that keeps us stuck and often creates psychological trauma. We have to learn how to hand over our maps (birth plans) at this gate so we can separate ourselves from the attachment of expectations and learn to create our own maps from our inner connection and intuition.

As doulas, we have seen how unfulfilled birth plans create disappointment, dissatisfaction, and trauma. It's human nature to set goals, and when they aren't reached, we feel a sense of loss. However, as doulas, we can say that it is very rare for any mother to achieve exactly what her birth plan states. Even if 99.9 percent of the birth plan is achieved miraculously (and most birth plans aren't fully met just by the nature of birth), but the laboring mom had the expectation that 100 percent would be achieved, she could experience disappointment and dissatisfaction in herself and her birth. This is why birth plans can be dangerous things if we don't hand them over the moment labor begins—they set us up to have a false sense of reality in birth.

We often counsel our clients to use their birth plan to mentally prepare, understand, and communicate birth wishes with others, but to then leave it at that. We ask that they understand that birth plans are idealized scenarios of what we would like to happen if everything goes perfectly. But it is also important to recognize that birth is messy, unpredictable, unplannable, uncontrollable and perfectly imperfect. To believe or hope otherwise may prove foolish. So, we encourage our families to make loose birth plans with loose expectations to minimize the pain of handing over the map when it is time. Failure to do so is the number-one reason we get stuck at this gate.

The Drive to Control

When the human desire to control our circumstances is balanced with a sense of flexibility and trust, it is healthy and helpful in birth. However, when control hardens the mind and heart, we start to work against the natural energy of labor and can create unnecessary complications for ourselves and our babies.

It's important to know that birth is an experience of flow and change. That means it isn't linear, solid, or rigid. So, our bodies, our emotions, our thoughts, and our expectations best serve us when they mimic this flexible nature of flow and change. Flexible emotions and thoughts mean an easier birth. Allowing ourselves to shift with change as labor shifts, all without fight or resistance ensures a much more pleasurable experience. The one thing that can disrupt flexibility like no other is anxious control energy.

When anxiety in the form of control enters our environment, it no longer feels okay to go with the flow. This is because control energy is rooted in the deep pain of feeling unsafe, which is a deeply disturbing feeling when we are as open and vulnerable as we are in pregnancy and birth. So, anxiety enters to help our egos rest assured that we won't be taken advantage of, overlooked, dismissed, or belittled while we are in this vulnerable state. When we start to anxiously control the situation, trust is thrown out the window, and we can find ourselves stuck at this gate.

It's important to really understand: the only thing we control in birth is *how* we react when our expectations are not met. Do we feel anxious and motivated to control more of our surroundings, or do we shrug it off and lean into deeper trust? This is a great question to ask in our daily lives and we should examine how we react to disappointment in general. The answer to this question will shed a lot of light on how control, disappointment, and anxiety may show up when labor doesn't go exactly your way.

A fun anecdote we tell our clients is that the Surprise Fairy shows up in every birth—no one comes out unscathed by her surprise dust. Some get a gentle misting of surprise in birth, and others get a soaking. As doulas, we've found that moms-to-be who have trust and control issues tend to get the biggest dusting. The moms-to-be who are more flexible tend to receive a gentler dustings of surprise. This is another motivation to work out *how* you react to surprise, especially unwanted surprise before labor begins.

A DOULA'S BIRTH STORY

Debbie was an immigrant from Bali who moved to the U.S. when she was two years old with her mother and her three sisters. She grew up hearing stories about Bali and life over there. So, when she became pregnant, she really wanted to have a different kind of birth than her mother experienced. She wanted to have an all-natural experience, not a C-section, which was how she was born. As she worked through this program and walked through the gates, she discovered that the main reason why she was born via C-section was that the doctor told her mother that she was too big to deliver vaginally. This later proved to be false because Debbie was a small 6 lbs., 10 oz at birth.

Debbie decided that this wasn't going to happen to her, and she created a rather rigid birth plan to have an all-natural vaginal birth. Seeing this as a red flag, I encouraged her to soften her expectations and even spent two hours going through other possible birth scenarios, including C-section, to help her open her mind to all possibilities of birth and detach herself from her expectations.

When Debbie's labor started, she confided in me that there was no way she was going to have a C-section. I could tell immediately that her resistance was playing a dangerous game, and from my experience, these types of women were the ones who ended up having C-sections.

She labored brilliantly for hours and the time came to push. The doctor told her if she didn't get the baby out in the next hour, she would need a C-section. Her fear of this prospect made her pain soar, and pushing was very slow going. I could see how much she was resisting the Gate of Expectations and how she just couldn't release her dream of having a vaginal birth. I looked her in the eye and said, "This is your last chance to birth your baby vaginally, but you have to surrender to this gate. You have to let go of control and be okay with getting a C-section."

At that moment, peace overcame her, and she said, "Yes. I'm done fighting. If it has to be a C-section, then so be it." In two more pushes, her baby was out, just as the C-section team arrived to take her to the OR. The moment she surrendered her expectation, she got what she really wanted!"

As witnessed by Alexandria Moran

This particular birth is such a great example of the power of letting go of our expectations. So many times in birth, we resist letting go and end up, causing ourselves complications and trauma. It's likely that if Debbie hadn't finally surrendered, she would have had the C-section and the emotional and psychological consequences of wondering, "What happened? Why couldn't I move through the gate?" Luckily, she surrendered just in the nick of time and got the outcome she wanted.

So much of birth and motherhood is about being flexible enough to let go . . . let go of the old, let go of the fear, let go of the shame, let go of the control, let go of the expectation, let go of the disappointment. When we let go in birth, energy flows through us. When we hold, resist, or control, we block that energy and create all kinds of physical, emotional, and psychological pain. We can work toward the ideal birth we want, but we must also be flexible enough to release our expectations of birth going our way. We have to let the experience be what it needs to be, without control or judgment.

The ultimate goal for all of us is to get to a point in our personal evolution where disappointment is something we can easily face, acknowledge, honor, and understand that control is something we can easily release. The Integration Practices at the end of this chapter are tools that have helped the most controlling and anxious moms find inner trust and flexibility in labor. We believe they can work for you too!

Understanding Our Wants vs. Needs

Most birth plans tell us and others what we *want* out of our birth. But they don't touch on what we actually need out of it—emotionally, spiritually, physically or psychologically. They definitely don't take into consideration what our babies need under their personal soul plan. That's because we often confuse our wants with our needs, and this is where disappointment can show up. Learning the difference can be a crucial step in allowing ourselves to surrender to the sacrifices of this gate.

So, let's talk about wants since we are probably more aware of our wants. We can define a *want* as a desire, wish, or hope as to *how* the birth unfolds (i.e., the circumstances and location, length of labor, level of intensity, what medical procedures will be performed or available, etc.). Wants are listed on our birth plans and are often idealized scenarios. Even if we don't write down an actual birth plan, we develop our wants through fantasizing, imagining, and daydreaming about our births. We ask ourselves, "What is my goal in birth?" We often answer with tangible answers like "a natural birth," "a healthy baby," or "a pain-free birth," and with the physical ways we believe we will achieve these goals like "birth at a birthing center," "birth with a midwife," "with an epidural," or "without medication,".

Now let's talk about *needs*. Needs are our emotional, psychological, and spiritual desires that are important to our evolution and welfare. They are expressed more as intentions than actions. For example, a birthing need would be, "I need to feel empowered and safe while I birth my baby" or "I need a calm atmosphere while I labor." These focus on feelings and energies rather than specific ways of achieving the desire.

But wants and needs can get muddled together, which makes it confusing to understand the difference. For example, we may say to ourselves, "I need to birth in a birthing center because that is the only way I will have an empowered birth." If we take the definitions from above, "birthing in a birthing center" is a want, not a need because it describes a physical circumstance. The need in this statement is to "have an empowered birth." The reason this distinction is important shows up when this mom can't birth in a birthing center due to a medical complication and must be in a hospital. If she has attached herself to her expectation of want, she will believe that she no longer can have an empowered birth outside of the birthing center, setting her labor up for disappointment from the get-go. However, if the mom shifts her focus to her need to "have an empowered birth," she will bring that attitude to whatever environment in which she is birthing and will more likely experience her birth as empowering.

Seeing "circumstances" as wants and "emotional experiences" as needs can help us sift through our personal expectations of birth. We often make the mistake of thinking that a circumstance is going to get us satisfaction, but it's really the emotional experience that will leave us feeling satisfied with our birth experience, no matter what happens circumstantially. This is what we as doulas really started to see as lacking in childbirth education. So many moms are prepared for circumstances, but they have no training on how to deal with their emotions when their expectations aren't meant. We personally believe this is why such a high number of women experience dissatisfaction with their birth experiences.

So a great thing to ask ourselves as we prepare for our births, create our birth plans and even deal with change as it comes up in labor is: "Will this [*fill in the blank decision*] bring me closer to the emotional experience I desire or further away from it?" The Integration Practices at the end of this chapter will help you unpack this tricky territory and get you to your core emotional experience that you need, want, and desire for your birth.

A DOULA'S BIRTH STORY

Adriene was a strong alpha female, a partner at her law firm, and very together. When planning for the birth of her first child, she did all the research and came up with a pretty extensive birth plan. She wanted to birth at the local birthing center, have peppermint essential oils, have a doula (me), and birth in the middle of the night. She was very specific on all the details, and I could tell she had spent a lot of time and energy thinking about this plan.

When she hired me, she was shocked that I wanted her to rework her birth plan, since she had spent so much time on it. But after learning about the gates and doing the Integration Practices in this book, she realized the value in reworking it. She created an Energetic Birth Plan right next to her original one, and she spent a lot of time focusing on the feelings she wanted to have in birth and how to face disappointment when it came up. I was surprised how much she dedicated herself to practicing the gates in pregnancy, at work, with colleagues with family members, whenever she could.

On the day of her labor, she felt very prepared and created a one-statement mantra to focus on throughout the labor. She wrote it on sticky notes all over the house and said it over and over to herself, "I want and need to feel empowered and strong throughout this labor, no matter what happens."

> Her labor progressed very quickly, and as we were getting ready to head to the birthing center, she got the urge to push. The midwife thought it was too early, so she had Adriene sit on the toilet to see if she needed to go to the bathroom. But sure enough, she was ready to push, and she almost had the baby in the toilet. I was so worried because this was the exact opposite of her birth plan! But she looked up to me and said, "I've never felt more empowered or strong as I do now! I got what I needed!"
>
> **Witnessed by Alexandria Moran**

Creating an Energetic Birth Plan

This may seem radical, but a great way to walk through this gate is to throw out your birth plan completely (all the circumstantial expectations) and rewrite it as an Energetic Birth Plan (based on your emotional, psychological, and spiritual needs). We've found that the moms who do this end up feeling much more empowered, satisfied, and happy about their birth experiences. Because at the end of the day, the what, where, and when are not up to us; the only thing we can control is *how* we feel in labor.

An Energetic Birth Plan (see Appendix I for an example) takes the list of all your wants and then asks the question, "What emotional experience am I trying to achieve?" Then all the circumstances are erased, and what is left is just the emotional experience you need to feel empowered in birth.

When we focus on the need, we can walk through the Gates of Transformation in a slightly more intuitive and introspective way. We don't get caught up in the how, but rather the energy we want to be in. In the example with Adriene, she could have been very disappointed by having her baby in the bathroom, rather than at the very expensive and lush birthing center as she had wanted. But because she spent most of her pregnancy and labor focusing on her Energetic Birth Plan, and the energy she wanted to be in, when things changed, like pushing on a toilet, rather than in a peppermint-scented bath, it didn't even faze her. There was no room for disappointment because she was so focused and committed to the energy of empowerment and strength despite the circumstance. Even months later, she felt grateful for the distinction because, without it, she was sure that she would have been very disappointed and maybe would have tried to sue the midwife for not getting her to the birthing center faster! What a difference this mental shift can make.

Another benefit of the Energetic Birth Plan is that it is something all members of the birth team can hold space for, especially when things go "wrong." When your birth partner knows that "feeling safe" or "having privacy" is your most important experience, they can better support you in achieving that. When birth partners try to make circumstances happen, their own feelings of frustration, anger, resentment, and disappointment may flare up and enter the birth space, because they can't control birth, either. They may feel responsible for what happens in labor. This is especially true if the birth partner is also the father and feels a deep drive to protect mama and baby from disappointment. But if the birth partner is freed from the responsibility of ensuring a particular circumstance, they can better hold that Divine Masculine space (see Chapter 6) and support their partner's needs more compassionately and without their own agenda. They become better birth partners.

Bottom line: When we are at peace because our needs are met, our babies are free to birth themselves with safety, peace, and love, even if we are in the back of a cramped taxi. When we feel our needs are being met, because we are meeting them with the emotional choices we are making, our babies feel supported as well. The Energetic Birth Plan ensures a space of love for our children to be born into—and that is the greatest gift we can give our newborns!

Babies Choose Their Birth Circumstances

We believe how a baby is born is part of their soul path and the foundation for their personality for the rest of their lives. This is the main reason that babies control the length and intensity of contractions (see also Chapter 7). The soul chooses its womb, its lineage, and its birth experience. Our children picked us as mothers, picked their birth experiences, and picked their birth complications as part of their path, their karma, and their soul story.

This is kind of amazing if we think about it because it takes a lot of the pressure off of us pregnant women to 'perform' in labor. When we realize that the baby is the one in control, then we can just be the vehicle for the unfolding journey. This is why when we get out of the baby's way, by going through the Gates of Transformation and releasing all the blocks that may hinder the baby's progress, we have easier births. But this doesn't mean that we are guaranteed to have birth go a certain way. If a baby needs to be born by C-section, to learn certain lessons this lifetime, nothing we can do will stop that, even if we flawlessly move through our gates. As we've said so many times before, birth is not in our control, and some find this perspective really comforting.

Our babies are destined to come into the world in their own unique way. As mothers, sacrificing our control and releasing expectations are great acts of service on their behalf. Being okay with whatever happens in birth and trusting that our baby will be born in the exact way it needs to for its own spiritual path is a bold act of unconditional love and motherhood. Creating an Energetic Birth Plan is a great way of creating a space where we are reminded of this powerful truth to allow our babies to be born in love.

How Past Trauma Can Block Us

The one thing that can make an Energetic Birth Plan feel impossible to achieve is unresolved trauma because it can make letting go of expectations and control really hard—maybe even feel life-threatening. When dealing with deep emotional pain, trauma, and PTSD, facing any of the gates can be extremely challenging, and a lot of resistance can come up. We've supported many women with trauma and have witnessed the courage, strength, and freedom from that trauma that they exhibit by walking through the Gates of Transformation.

This is why it's important to know that we don't have to be 100 percent healed of our traumas before the baby comes and we don't know any woman who is. The act of labor allows us to heal the trauma the moment we surrender to a gate's sacrifice. Nowhere else in life do we get to have this level of escalated healing. The secret to embracing this opportunity is in understanding our traumas so we can see them for what they are and recognize when they show up in labor or birth. Then we can walk through the gate to heal ourselves simultaneously.

What Is Trauma?

According to *Psychology Today*, trauma is a natural response of the nervous system when we experience or perceive something life-threatening, to ourselves or others. It affects the emotional, spiritual, mental, physical, and social parts of our lives. When trauma isn't processed out of the nervous system, it can turn into PTSD where the body doesn't realize it is no longer in that life-threatening experience and behaves as if the trauma were still occurring.

In plain English, trauma is the thing that happens to us when something really intense occurs, and the body interprets the experience as a life-or-death crisis. It can happen just once like a car accident or be an on going, prolonged series of events like childhood sexual abuse. But the body feels so threatened that the experience ends up staying in our myofascial tissues, rather than being released, the way that wild animals shake to release the possibility of residual trauma.

Wherever a particular trauma falls on the scale of perceived severity, it usually affects us on many levels—emotional, cognitive, physical, spiritual, and social. It can affect how we process our thoughts and even affect our ability to make sound decisions. It can trap emotions in a loop (of fear or shame or anger, for example) and make it feel impossible to release. It can get stuck in our physical bodies and affect our digestion, immunity, sleep patterns, and even stamina. It also affects us on the spiritual level, perhaps negatively coloring our view of the world, our belief systems, and our meaning in life. Finally, trauma can affect our social interactions and can cause us to withdraw and distance ourselves from loved ones or engage in risky behavior with strangers. This is how trauma can cause all sorts of problems in our daily lives.

However, it is important to understand that trauma isn't only a psychological or mental block that we can just "get over," although sometimes we feel like we just should. It's a whole-system disruption, which is why it can take time to heal, even with lots of support and understanding. So, as you read this book, if any trauma shows up for you, allow yourself deep compassion if you can. Reach out to a friend, or better yet, a therapist, healer, or professional to help you move through the trauma if you are ready. As we said before, you don't have to be healed to labor like a goddess; you just have to be willing to look at it.

Ways Trauma Can Show Up in Birth

This next section may be a bit triggering, but we invite you to read it with an open heart. We feel it is important to illustrate the ways we, as doulas, have seen trauma show up in the birth space, because more often than not, it is very alarming for the laboring woman when she doesn't expect it. We hope this section will help you understand when and how trauma can show up in birth and help you feel better prepared should it show up in your labor. Then, if it does, you can recognize it for what it is, and hopefully, place it to the side while you continue laboring. We've seen firsthand what happens when women get lost in unresolved trauma and run the risk of further traumatizing themselves, so this section is just a friendly hello to the unexpected ways trauma can show up in birth.

Traumatic Shame

We've already discussed shame in the previous chapter, but here we want to talk about traumatic shame, which is shame created by a traumatic incident that has gotten stuck in a trigger/reaction loop. The problem with this is that we often get so wrapped up in reacting to it that we don't see it for what it is—old shame resurfacing.

The easiest way to recognize traumatic shame is that it doesn't build gradually, but hits us fast and hard, like a train. It also is so painful that we desperately grasp at whatever coping mechanisms are available to avoid, distance ourselves, or numb ourselves to it. Traumatic shame also immediately puts us right back into the moment, age, and mental state that we were in when we first felt victimized by the trauma. Once we come out of it, the shame spiral continues because we feel ashamed about how we just reacted. So, it's shame on top of shame on top of shame.

A DOULA'S BIRTH STORY

Dina was a smart, accomplished woman and first-time mom. She was very nervous about giving birth and having her mother in the birth room. After many sessions together, she opened up to me that her mother was verbally abusive and made her feel like a little kid. Dina was really afraid of her mother being at her labor and didn't want her energy there. To help remedy the situation, I suggested that she not call her mother until after the baby was born to ensure that she would have the birth experience she wanted. Dina loved the idea and decided to do just that.

Her birth day came upon us, and Dina labored like a goddess, bravely walking through each and every gate. I could see her surrender and willingness to transform into a mother. Everything was moving beautifully until her mother walked through the door, upset that she hadn't been called when Dina went into labor. She said to Dina, "I don't know how you thought you could birth this baby on your own. I'm your mother, and I know you. You just can't do it without me."

I then watched this very strong and capable laboring woman deflate down into the mentality and physicality of a five-year-old. I've never seen anything like it. She was having a traumatic response to her mother. Her voice changed into a little girl's, her body language became passive, and she literally looked defeated as her mother took charge of the room, ordering around medical staff and complaining about the quality of the linens. This strong goddess, who was laboring not more than a minute ago, now appeared to be a pregnant child—and debilitated by shame. Her labor became difficult as her body and mind were no longer in it and she needed to have a C-section to get her baby out safely.

After surgery, Dina sobbed. I thought it was because she had to have surgery, but I discovered she was just embarrassed by what happened. She was now compounding her own shame on top of her traumatic shame. It broke my heart. But on the bright side, it was a wake-up call for Dina to finally deal with her past trauma, and she did. Her second birth was empowering and inspiring, even though her mother was there, acting the same way as the first time! Nothing had changed except for Dina! It's amazing what can happen when we face our traumas."

As witnessed by Alexandria Moran

Traumatic shame can come from a wide range of experiences, some obvious and some less so: a rough pelvic or medical exam, unwelcome or aggressive sex, saying yes when wanting to say no, physical abuse and violence, sexual abuse, molestation, manipulation, rape, victimization, invalidation, feeling discredited or undermined, enslavement, being a victim of power abuse, and many more. So, it is important to realize that even if we were lucky enough to never have had a violent or abusive event in our lives, we still could have trauma from unexpected sources. Just remember that the process of dealing with our trauma as it gets triggered, recognizing that it is an old story that the body is just reliving, and focusing on a new story is the key to getting through labor. Then at a later time, we can focus on the long-term work of healing.

As Complications

We all dream of a complication-free birth, but it is just a dream. Every birth gets a visit from the Surprise Fairy who sprinkles a little bit of surprise on each labor. Sometimes she sprinkles a dusting of surprise, and sometimes it is an avalanche. But one thing's for certain: surprise happens in birth. Add trauma to the mix, and we've got ourselves a unique set of complication opportunities.

Because both birth and trauma are such physical experiences, it is only logical to surmise that the two will collide in labor and usually not for the benefit of mom and baby. In most of the births we've seen, unexplained complications are usually later understood as resistance to old trauma from the past. A doula trick is to look for resistance to trauma when labor slows (e.g., baby won't turn, contractions stop completely, or a whole slew of other mysterious happenings). We often find if we can just start talking about the trauma, allowing it to be seen and heard, the labor complications disappear. It's as if the complications make us stop and pay attention to something that needs to be acknowledged first before labor can continue. And in our experience, this is often the case.

A DOULA'S BIRTH STORY

Jessica was a high-risk mom with hypertension and other medical concerns. She knew that natural birth wasn't in the cards, so when she went into labor, we went to the hospital sooner than normal to ensure everything was okay with mom and baby. She got an epidural pretty soon after and was doing really well. She even fell asleep. As her doula, I left her husband in the room with her and excused myself to refresh, eat, and stretch my legs. I was gone for about 30 minutes, and when I returned to the room, Jessica was all alone sobbing. Her husband had gone to the bathroom, and when Jessica woke up, she was all alone in a dark hospital room in the middle of the night, and she couldn't feel her legs.

I only later learned that she started to have flashbacks to a date rape experience in college when she also couldn't move in a dark room. She hadn't thought about that experience in 10 years. Her trauma was triggered, and even though her body was relaxed from the epidural, her emotions skyrocketed. She visibly calmed down, and I massaged her head, but she refused to talk about it. Within a few minutes, all the machine bells and alarms were blasting. Her blood pressure soared, and she was carted off for an emergency C-section faster than I could blink. I would like to believe that if she had been able to talk about the trauma, she might have been able to calm her nervous system and her blood pressure and maybe even avoid the emergency complication. Later she told me that she was happy to have the C-section because she was able to get out of that painful trauma memory much faster, as she couldn't shake it herself.

As witnessed by Alexandria Moran

As Resistance to the Gates

This is the most common way we see trauma show up in birth: resistance. Resistance is a physical, emotional, psychological, and sometimes spiritual unwillingness to face the sacrifice being asked of us in labor.

Sometimes we physically resist by tightening our bodies, pulling back, holding in. We've witnessed many laboring women being asked to hold their babies in until a doctor is present for delivery, which is a physical form of resisting the Gate of Intentional Surrender (see Chapter 8). Or, if we have had a traumatic tear in a previous birth, we may physically resist the pushing stage out of fear of re-experiencing that trauma. Or if we fear a sexual re-traumatizing, we may resist our baby coming down the birth canal and touching those organs. Sometimes, in these cases, epidurals can be the best way to numb the physical sensation and help us to not resist physically.

We also can emotionally and cognitively resist the Gates of Transformation. We've talked extensively about how we do that with fear and shame, and we will continue to go through many more emotions of resistance in the remaining chapters. But what is important to note here is how our unwillingness to feel our own emotions can create resistance in our space and affect our labors.

Finally, we can resist the spiritual transformation from Maiden-to-Mother that happens in labor. This is more of an individual experience because spirituality is very different for each of us. But when we resist, it can feel like a refusal to level up, to grow, to expand consciousness and step into a new role. We might feel victimized when we resist because birth, unfortunately, doesn't wait for our permission to push us into motherhood. So, we have to learn to ride the wave, just like we learn to ride the waves of our contractions.

However we resist, one thing is certain: resistance causes trauma in birth. If you take one thing away from this book, let it be to surrender fully to the life force that is asking you to walk through the Gates of Transformation. The moment we resist a gate or refuse to walk through, we risk inserting trauma into our birth story. When we have trauma, we have stuck energy that needs to be healed. It also makes it more difficult to fully transition into motherhood and can complicate postpartum recovery, bonding with baby, and adjustment to our new lives in the fourth trimester. So we insist . . . please don't resist. Allow yourself to soften into the mold birth wants for you.

How to Walk Through the Gate of Expectations

The one thing trauma needs more than anything else is to be witnessed with compassion by the person who is experiencing it. This is a tall order because we can so easily get lost in our trauma that we get trapped in the victimization of a past experience. Being able to see the traumatized parts of ourselves as little children who need to be heard, acknowledged, and loved is often the last thing that interests us.

But in our experience, this is one of the best ways to regain sovereignty over trauma so we can actually begin the journey into healing. Getting professional support is a really powerful way to do just that. There are a wide variety of healers, therapists, and counselors specializing in healing trauma, not to mention a wide variety of techniques such as psychotherapy, equine therapy, EFT, EMDR, shaman healing, womb work, art therapy, and movement. We invite you to do some research and invest in a practitioner you connect with and trust. Nothing is more precious than your own wellbeing, and we all deserve an amazing life, especially after trauma!

Integration Practices

The following practices are intended to help you integrate the information of this chapter and apply it to your life now, so you can walk through the Gate of Expectations with trust and consciousness while in labor! Take your time going through the practices that resonate the most with you and feel free to do them as often as you'd like.

Self-Love Activity: Energetic Birth Plan

One of the best ways to prepare for this gate is to come face to face with your expectations about birth through this extensive Energetic Birth Plan process. Here you will fill out the table below. See Appendix I for an example from one of the author's births.

1. First, write out the overall energetic intention you want for your birth from the viewpoint of spiritual growth.
2. Next, write out the circumstances you want at the birth (the how, what, where, when).
3. Then, describe the energy and emotional experience you need to have (feelings and atmosphere) to feel fulfilled and satisfied with your birth.
4. Next, describe, the worst-case scenario (usually the opposite to the circumstances you prefer)
5. Finally, write out positive reactions you can choose to have to the worst-case scenario that maintains your energetic intention.

ENERGETIC BIRTH PLAN

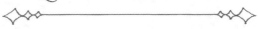

MY ENERGETIC INTENTIONS FOR MY BIRTH:	THE CIRCUMSTANCES I PREFER AND/OR WANT TO HAPPEN:	THE ENERGY AND EMOTIONAL EXPERIENCE I NEED:	THE WORST-CASE SCENARIO THAT COULD HAPPEN:	SHOULD THE WORST HAPPEN, WHAT I CAN DO TO UPHOLD MY INTENTION:
Example: I intend to feel calm, safe and empowered throughout my labor and delivery.	*Example:* An epidural when I arrive as soon as I get into active labor.	*Example:* I emotionally need to feel safe and not overwhelmed by past sexual trauma. I need my sex organs numb.	*Example:* I can't have an epidural or it doesn't work and my sexual trauma is retriggered. I end up feeling victimized and powerless.	*Example:* I can choose to recognize my baby needs to be born this way and I can lean on my birth partner for support. I can tell myself I am safe, even if I feel triggered.

Once you create this chart for yourself, have your birth partner do one, too. Yours might be more baby-focused, and your partner might be more you-focused. It's important to have these conversations because the last thing you want is a conflict in labor that you haven't discussed ahead of time. If everyone is on the same page as to what your wants are and what your needs are, the birth team will be in alignment with making decisions based on your emotional needs as circumstances change and surprises come up. After completing this chart, record the following:

- What are the positive recurring words of intention? These will be the words that show up the most frequently. In the example above: "safe" and "calm"
- Do some journaling to reflect on which Gates of Transformation stand out and could use some more work
- Write a statement of commitment to uphold your Energetic Birth Plan
- Expand on your Energetic Birth Intention
- Share this with your birth team

SELF-LOVE ACTIVITY: COLLAGE YOUR SAFE SPACE

After completing the exercise above, a great way to really integrate the energy of your Energetic Birth Plan is to allow your creative side to take over with some birth art. In this self-love exploration, you can collect images from magazines, or Pinterest, or even create your own art to capture the feeling, atmosphere, and energy of your personal safe space. Once you've collected all the images, print and cut them out to create a collage on a poster board. This will be a visual representation of the energy you want to have in your birth space. You can even bring it to your birth room to inspire you and remind your birth team of your intentions.

INNER EXPLORATION JOURNAL PROMPTS

The following journal prompts are for you to explore and uncover the different challenges of this gate. The practice of journaling can be deeply healing and enlightening, so we encourage you to spend some time reading over the prompts to see which ones resonate with you. Look back at these often. You might notice that different journal prompts resonate at different times.

Releasing Expectations

- What are some of my expectations that are difficult to release?
- How do I usually deal with disappointment?
- What can I do to support myself when disappointment shows up in birth?
- How does my birth partner deal with disappointment?
- How can my birth partner support me through this gate?

Asking for Help

- Do I have a difficult time asking for help? Why or why not?
- How do I feel when others help me?
- What do I believe it says about my character if I ask for or receive help?
- Do I prefer to do everything on my own? If so, why?

- In what ways have I already asked for help?
- What areas of pregnancy, labor, or postpartum can I ask for more help?

Issues With Trust

- Do I trust easily? Why or why not?
- Do I trust my body completely? Why or why not?
- Do I trust my baby completely? Why or why not?
- Can I trust that my baby's birth will be exactly what he/she needs? Why or why not?
- How can I improve my ability to trust now, in pregnancy?
- What do I need to feel safe enough to trust? Can I create this sense at my birth?

Unpacking Trauma

- Do I have any known trauma from my past that I can deal with now?
- What happens if an unknown or hidden trauma pops up for me while I am laboring?
- Who can I reach out to for additional support?

GODDESS RITUAL: PACK AND UNPACK YOUR BIRTH BAG

This is a very practical yet symbolic ritual that can shed light on your unconscious expectations. This can be a very powerful tool in understanding the differences between your wants and needs in birth. Do this on your own or with your birth partner.

What You Need:

- Overnight bag
- Items to bring to your birth

What to Do:

Pack one bag with everything that you want to bring into your birth room. Examples include a robe to labor in, essential oils, snacks, clean underwear, toiletries, or clothes for the baby. Once you have the whole bag packed, unpack it, imagining that you are unpacking your bag on your birth day. Hold each item for 5–10 seconds and reflect on how each item makes you feel. Does it stir up emotion? Do you need it? Do you want it? Does it bring you comfort? Does it align with your Energetic Birth Plan? You may find that there are items you don't really want but thought you needed and there might be items you have totally forgotten about. Let this little preparation ritual take you into your true wants and needs for preparing for birth.

GODDESS RITUAL: MAIDEN-TO-MOTHER AFFIRMATION

Say the following affirmation as often as you like aloud, quietly or as a mantra over and over again as you transition from Maiden-to-Mother. Place your hands over your solar plexus chakra and say: *"I release the need to fight or control my circumstances. I easily and freely go with the natural flow of pregnancy and labor and I hold the intention of love for myself and my baby."*

THRESHOLD MEDITATION

In this meditation, you'll go on a short journey through the Gate of Expectations to enter into greater trust in the divine unfolding. This is a perfect meditation if you are struggling to release control and expectations. This practice can be done after each journal prompt or daily until you feel complete in your transition. It is also a great meditation to put on during labor when those moments of control or victimization show up. Go to www.laborlikeagoddess.com to download it.

Final Thoughts

Walking through this gate is a matter of release and acceptance: releasing control, releasing expectations, and releasing old trauma imprints and accepting the natural unfolding of the birth experience and your baby's divine plan. Being able to do this is a fiercely feminine energy, but if we have trauma or control issues in our space, it can be a rather challenging gate. To be willing to release expectations and accept what is, we have to feel safe and allow ourselves to be vulnerable. We hope that this chapter has inspired you to focus your emotional and mental energies on a sense of empowerment despite the surprise circumstances that may, and will, show up in your birth. We believe you can do it!

~ CHAPTER V ~

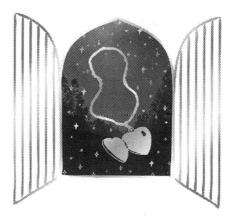

THE GATE
OF EMBODIMENT
BECOMING PRESENT

I have worshipped woman as the living embodiment of the spirit of service and sacrifice.

—*Mahatma Gandhi*

*L*earning how to trust her heart to find her way was a bit clunky at first. She had never needed to trust this deeply or listen so intuitively for direction. But as she turned inward, she realized how easy it was to find her way in the darkness, and that she had an internal compass that had been there all along. She just couldn't access it when she was fixated on the map. She laughed at herself for her naivety and felt blessed to have found this new part of herself. She was able to move so much quicker and easier with this internal compass than when she was relying on someone else's directions.

And, before she knew it, she came upon a fourth gate, just like the others, big, iron-clad and enchanted. And she knocked.

A fourth Gatekeeper appeared, just as old, just as haggish as the others, asking what business the Maiden Goddess had knocking on her door.

"I long to become a mother. I wish to go to the Underworld," the Maiden Goddess replied with more authority in her voice than she'd had at any of the previous gates.

"Ah, yes, I see," said the Gatekeeper. "Then you will need to go through this gate."

"Yes, I know, I know," the Maiden Goddess said, "So what must I give you to receive passage?"

"It's not what you give me, my dear. It is what I give you. If you accept my gift, I will open the gate. This is the sacrifice required."

"A gift? You are giving me a gift? That doesn't seem like such a sacrifice," the Maiden Goddess exclaimed. "Yes, I agree!"

The old Gatekeeper handed the Maiden Goddess a beautiful iron locket, and she could see it was enchanted. "What a lovely gift," she thought . . . That was until she felt the weight of the locket which hung like an anchor around her neck. This was indeed not a gift but the biggest sacrifice yet. She began to cry and scream from the agony of it. "What is this?" she demanded.

"This is the locket of embodiment," the Gatekeeper said. "It forces you to be present with all your thoughts, emotions, and ideas. It grounds your soul into your body, and you are not able to escape, hide, or numb yourself. You will need to learn to accept yourself fully and be fully present."

When the Maiden Goddess heard this, she was instantly enraged, and at that moment became aware of how much she did indeed avoid, numb, and disassociate in everyday life. "How painful it is to face all of myself," she thought.

But just like with the previous gates, she told herself that if this were the price of becoming a mother, she would pay it, for she wanted nothing more.

Despite her resistance to being embodied, she said to herself, "I will no longer fear or avoid my truth, because it is me and always has been. I now embrace and embody my whole self—the good, the bad, and the ugly. I fully accept myself, and I lean in with love. Bring on the embodiment!"

With her acceptance, the gate flung open, and the Maiden Goddess felt her heart expand in a million different directions. She felt a deep sense of connection to herself and to every mother who came before her. She felt her baby, her beloved, and everyone she had ever loved breathing through her heart space. At that moment, she realized her self-acceptance had not only opened this gate, but also the invisible gates and barriers around her heart. Ironically, she found the greatest freedom when she couldn't escape.

The Gift of the Locket

What a strange gate this is. The Gate of Embodiment is unlike the ones that have come before, because this time the Maiden Goddess *receives* a gift—the Locket of Embodiment. Choosing to wear this *gift* becomes her greatest sacrifice because being fully embodied during birth often feels more like a curse than a gift. When the intensity of emotion and physical sensation kicks in during labor, the desire to disassociate, numb, avoid, or run away can sound like sweet relief. And it very well should, because as humans it is hard to be in our bodies when experiencing transformation. It's painful!

From a spiritual standpoint, most of us walk around with our souls floating just above our heads while our faces are in our phones rather than allowing our souls to properly anchor into our heart chakras. The soul is literally outside of the body most of the time. This is the definition of being *dis-embodied,* which has both its benefits and drawbacks, depending upon the circumstance. Don't believe us? Well, ask yourself: Have you ever gotten into your car, zoned out, and somehow ended up at your destination 20 minutes later, not knowing how you got there? Yes? Well, that is the perfect example of being disembodied. It's like the soul pops up and out, the body goes on autopilot, and we just aren't really there. We are not present. Now imagine a child running out into the street right in front of you while you are driving on autopilot. If we are lucky, the soul jolts back into the body to make a lifesaving decision to brake. Most of us have experienced that jolting adrenaline rush at one time or another when the soul suddenly comes back into the body. This is the jolt that comes from putting on that locket—from choosing embodiment.

We don't just disembody when we are driving, we also do it when we watch TV, drink alcohol, do drugs, or mindlessly eat a whole box of Oreos in one sitting. Basically, whenever we are zoned out, or numb, to the moment, we are not in our bodies. Some call it "mindlessness." Others call it "not being present" or a "lack of awareness." Whatever the term, when we "check out," the physical body automatically switches to autopilot, making decisions based on primal impulses or old habits—which is how all those Oreos mysteriously disappear. It's easy to see how being disembodied can quickly derail our health, our goals, and our intentions for life because no one's home.

But disembodiment can also be a helpful, valid coping mechanism too—and one of the most effective ways of taking the edge off of life or coping with painful experiences. Leaving the body can give us the mental and emotional break we need from dealing with life so we can rest and reset. Perhaps this is why bars and reality TV are so popular in modern-day culture—they give us full permission to disembody.

In the case of a traumatic or violent event, leaving the body can be a lifesaver. What medicine calls "shock," we describe as "the soul leaving the body temporarily." This happens all the time with car accidents, sudden loss, abuse, or violent acts. Victims of these experiences often describe a moment where they are unaware of being in their body but instead experience themselves floating above the situation.

From a spiritual perspective, we understand the soul uses disembodiment to help lessen the physical experience of pain, trauma, shock, grief, etc.—a powerful coping mechanism which allows us to focus on the physical trauma. When the danger has passed, and the body feels safe again, the soul returns with those traumatized emotional and psychological parts to be dealt with and healed. This is known and experienced as PTSD (post-traumatic stress disorder)—where an old traumatic event feels emotionally and psychologically like it is occurring in the present moment. And in a way, it is because the body hasn't yet dealt with the emotional and psychological trauma because it wasn't there to be dealt with until now.

When the soul is trying to re-embody the unprocessed trauma, it can feel overwhelmingly emotionally painful, scary, and confusing. The Maiden Goddess comes face to face with these feelings when she puts on the locket and realizes how much unprocessed emotion is waiting for her attention to be healed.

This same realization happens in every birth. As mentioned earlier in the book, birth is our spirit's chance to bundle all the unresolved pain together and push it through for healing. So, when we choose to put on the Locket of Embodiment, it's important to know that the soul is returning with all of that unprocessed pain and trauma to be healed. This is why this locket can feel more like a curse than a gift if we don't understand what our souls are trying to do for us. But even if we don't have a ton of unprocessed pain or trauma to heal, just wearing the locket is painful in itself.

Being Embodied Can Feel Painful

Let's face it, just being human is often a painful, emotional, confusing, and difficult experience. It takes a tremendous amount of courage to live this so-called life, and we don't always have the energy, wisdom, tools, or motivation to face every challenge in every moment with perfect clarity and power. This is why it is so easy for us as modern humans to be disembodied. We are master procrastinators, connoisseurs of pain avoidance. It's so much easier to zone out to *Keeping Up with The Kardashians* than to have that honest and possibly divisive conversation with our spouse.

It's human nature to avoid pain, especially emotional pain. So we zone out. We numb. We avoid. We distract. We disassociate. We actively engage in activities that keep us out of our bodies, so we don't have to feel all the feels, hear the intuition, make the tough calls and face the pain we so desperately want to avoid. So, it is only natural to want to disembody when we go through labor too. Who wants to feel all *that*? Wouldn't it be great to just leave our bodies and eight hours later a baby appears? Most of us, including the Maiden Goddess, would probably say yes! And with modern-day surgery and technology to numb pain, we have the option to have a relatively "painless" birth experience—something our grandmothers and great grandmothers could only dream about.

But here's the thing. . . even with our best efforts to avoid pain during delivery, no one is free from the pain of transformation from Maiden-to-Mother—not physically, emotionally, mentally, or spiritually. To convince ourselves otherwise actually sets us up for greater emotional trauma, not to mention disappointment as well. Transformation and growth just can't happen without pain. Each hand washes the other. That is why they are called "growing pains."

Pain is a catalyst for transformation here to teach us endurance, perseverance, and fortitude—lessons that can't be learned and integrated effectively when we are not in the body (we'll explore how we can transform the pain in Chapter 7). This is another reason why walking through the

Gate of Embodiment is so important in creating strong foundations and resilience in motherhood. We've noticed in our work as doulas, that the moms who have a hard time wearing the locket—being present and facing their own gates in pregnancy and labor—find themselves struggling more in postpartum and often have fussier babies. Witnessing this phenomenon has made it clear to us that no one comes through the transition without walking through this gate, and those who willingly embody, even when it is painful, seem to experience a more peaceful transition than those who resist the sacrifice.

Gift vs. Sacrifice

Embodiment *is* a sacrifice, but it can also be reframed as a blessing—the gift the Gatekeeper wants us to see it as. We've already mentioned how wearing the locket is a chance to heal all the unprocessed trauma, so we don't develop PTSD or worse, manifest the same lessons over and over again. That is a big gift. But the other gift is that we are learning how to fully accept ourselves by choosing to feel and face the parts we so often run away from. Which can be, well, emotionally, and psychologically painful. But when we face the darkness, we also get to experience our lightness. But we have to choose to feel it all—shame, fear, pain, surrender, mini-deaths, grief, loss, sadness—and in doing so we get rewarded with the feelings of euphoria, pure bliss, indescribable empowerment, joy, victory, accomplishment, satisfaction, deep connection, and intimacy. These amazing feelings are especially amplified after birth.

Numbing any part of our transition from Maiden-to-Mother dampens both pain and pleasure. And reducing pleasure in birth does us a great disservice because pleasure is one of the best and easiest ways to get embodied and experience empowerment. Later in the chapter, we'll dive into this, but for now, just reflect on how easy it is to be fully present when experiencing pleasure like great sex or a favorite spa treatment versus how easy it is to run away from life at the end of a bad day or while going through a breakup. In birth, it is the same—when we numb our pain, we unfortunately also numb our pleasure, making it more difficult to be embodied and transform.

Science is starting to research and confirm this notion as it relates to birth. The National Center for Biotechnology Information found a significant increase in oxytocin levels (the love and pleasure hormone) in moms who did not have an epidural versus those who did. It appears that the physical numbing of the body reduced the availability of the pleasure hormone in women. This is a small and preliminary study, but it does speak to the idea that numbing on any level numbs the entire experience.

When we look at embodiment in birth as a gift, we can see that being present to the entire experience of birth offers us a truly once-in-a-lifetime opportunity to transform and fundamentally shift our understanding of life. We are changed on all levels of the self—mind, body, and spirit—in a way that lasts for a lifetime because all three were present and accounted for. Through this, we are gifted spiritual wisdom and emotional understanding that prepares us for the patience and compassion required in child-rearing, and we develop the courage and fortitude to face all challenges of motherhood with fierce confidence and self-love.

The irony is what the Maiden Goddess learns after walking through this gate—freedom comes when we can't escape. The *empowered birth* that so many seek is only possible when allowing ourselves to feel all our feelings, including disempowerment. We must be present in birth, steer the ship, make the decisions, and face the fears to really find empowerment and satisfaction. The physical body alone cannot facilitate empowerment when it is running on autopilot. The soul must be present to fully transition from Maiden-to-Mother.

Baby's First Act of Embodiment

If we haven't spelled it out already, embodiment is the "bringing of the spirit/soul/essence INTO the physical body—the union of the physical with the spiritual." On a very obvious level, that is exactly what birth is—a baby's soul merging into its physical body as they debut into the world. Heaven coming to Earth. Spiritual meeting physical. If we are confused as to what embodiment really is, we can look to our babies to teach us the way. Babies are some of the most embodied beings in the world with their fierce curiosity, intense sensuality, and awareness of the world through their limited scope of view. They feel and welcome all their emotions, sensations, and experiences—which allows them to grow and transform at an incredible rate. It's clear from watching a baby that embodiment facilitates transformation.

As mothers, we get the opportunity to support our child's first physical, emotional, and spiritual debut into the world by leading through example. When we choose embodiment during labor and delivery, we get to send the message to our babies, "It is safe to be embodied here. Look I'm doing it too. I'm right here with you. You are not alone. Let's do this together." It's a powerful motherly act of support, love, and encouragement for these spirit babies to permanently move into their new homes—their physical bodies.

Over the last three decades, the field of pre- and perinatal psychology research has made some amazing discoveries around the effects and imprints a baby's birth has on its sense of safety, self-worth, belonging and capacity to have healthy relationships based on love, empathy, and trust. Current research suggests that a mother's emotional state and that of her unborn child are far more closely related before and during birth than was previously thought[6]. New research[7] studying the effects of the birth experience on a person's baseline psychology is coming out each year, and it's becoming clear that our energy and intention as laboring women affects our babies in profound and life-altering ways.

On a physical level, this plays out in a more obvious and immediate way. Pregnant women with high levels of cortisol—a hormone that's considered an indicator of stress—are at greater risk for health complications with their babies including early and late births, low birth weight, and difficulty breathing at birth, all of which can result in low Apgar scores, a common measure that rates newborn health. If stress can have this kind of measurable effect on babies, imagine what the power of love can do. We believe modern research and ancient wisdom agree—the more lovingly embodied we are as mothers in labor, the healthier our children.

Embodiment Through Love

As doulas, we have witnessed firsthand how powerful *love* can be as a catalyst for embodiment, surrender, and transformation. We can credit much of the natural availability of love in labor to the hormone called oxytocin, aptly nicknamed the "love hormone." This hormone is at its highest levels when we are pregnant and giving birth. As the baby descends the birth canal, the mom gets flooded with more and more oxytocin. Baby simultaneously experiences greater amounts of oxytocin, putting them in emotional and hormonal resonance with mom. When oxytocin is allowed to flow uninterrupted within mom (meaning naturally and without drug interference), her brainwaves enter a theta state, and a deeply spiritual or meditative experience overtakes her. We call it a "love trance" and have noticed it is so much easier for laboring moms to move through the gates when in this trance. Perhaps because embodiment through love helps us soar through the gates.

Intentionally increasing our oxytocin levels during labor is a great way to get us into that love trance and avoid the temptation to disembody. As doulas, we often encourage as much oxytocin release as possible in labor through pleasure, visualization, and intimacy with a partner as a way to improve the embodiment for mom and baby. We've found that the more embodied a mom is and the calmer a baby is when born, the easier it is to breastfeed initially and the deeper the connection to the spiritual changes that have occurred. All of this results in faster recovery after birth for both mom and baby. So, it's not hard to see why embodiment is a preferred energetic space to be in when possible for labor and delivery.

We believe a birth full of empowerment, freedom, love, and strength simply can't happen without embodiment. There has to be a loving willingness to *labor like a goddess*, which means there has to be a loving willingness to be 100 percent present throughout labor, for every contraction, for every emotion, for every thought, for every surprise, and for every sensation. But real talk here: when are we ever truly 100 percent present? The answer: whenever we experience pleasure like kissing, laughing with friends, sex, shopping, indulging in our favorite dessert, or any other activity that produces oxytocin in the body. That's because pleasure = oxytocin = embodiment = more oxytocin = more embodiment = more pleasure.

But the nemeses of oxytocin? Fear, shame, and resistance. This is why we must learn to walk through the first three Gates of Transformation (see Chapters 2–4) before stepping into embodiment. We must learn how to face our fears, shames, and control issues so embodiment will feel like the gift it is meant to be.

It's also great to know that as we cross each gate, the body gets a dose of oxytocin, which affects the reward centers in the brain. That means we get to feel on a hormonal level the benefits of sacrifice, and it makes it that much easier for us to embody when the time comes. Like the Maiden Goddess, we know that reward is on the other side of embodiment even if pain is part of the journey. This is true even if we keep walking through a particular gate over and over and over again. Each time we get a deeper and deeper dose of that reward magic.

Choosing Conscious Embodiment

Here we would like to add a word of warning about embodying before learning to walk through the first three gates. Because embodiment requires us to feel ourselves fully, if we embody irresponsibly, we can end up creating unnecessary pain, suffering, or even trauma for ourselves. Being faced with great fears or shames, and having no understanding of how to deal with them, can be catastrophic to the Maiden-to-Mother journey. Just imagine what the Maiden Goddess would feel like if the first gate was the Gate of Embodiment and she had no experience or history with the previous gates. This is why we want to go through the gates that deal with fear, shame, and expectations first, while in pregnancy, so we have the tools and resources to face these feelings when they come up while we are embodied in labor.

If we have been doing the work in pregnancy and feel ready to embody with consciousness, we can start to practice what it means to embody every day. We can start to choose to feel it all and intentionally sit with discomfort, without avoiding or numbing it. If a gate shows up to be crossed again, we can practice crossing it with those lockets on. Learning to do this compassionately in pregnancy makes embodiment in labor so much easier. It becomes second nature and sets us up for blessings. For more insight on how to do this, check out the Integration Practices at the end of this chapter.

A DOULA'S BIRTH STORY

The clock is huge! I hadn't noticed it until now. A giant digital clock, right there, perfectly placed across the room. Why is it so big? My contractions are about two minutes apart, getting close to one minute. I'm really starting to feel the pressure. Everyone says that labor is painful, and it is, but it's really that pressure. That feeling of something pushing its way out. It needs to come out. "Ugh, I need to get out of my head." The thoughts, "My baby girl, is descending, she is working so hard to meet me. But gosh, I'm tired. I'm ready for this to be over. I wonder what she will be like? Will she look like my husband or me? I bet she looks just like her sister . . . Ugh, this pressure. It's making me be here now. I want to keep thinking about what tomorrow looks like. I think my mom is coming by. I wonder who else will come and visit. The weather is going to be really nice tomorrow, they will have an easy drive. I don't want to be here." This is all going through my head, I am moving into transition, I am ready to start pushing, and all I want to do is NOT BE HERE. I want to be in the future. God, that clock is huge—12:45, 12:49, 12:53. I'm focused on the clock. It's keeping me here. Every time I move my mind to the thought of tomorrow, time slows down. The moment lingers. I am in more pain—12:58. I need to start pushing. This baby is ready to come. The clock, that giant clock. Keeping me here. Another contraction . . . I am focused on. I am here. I don't need to know about tomorrow, the only thing that matters is right now . . . 13:03 another push and I roar. I roar like a lioness. I feel my body, I feel my spirit. I am in this moment . . . 13:10. I push through my last contraction. I am here, my daughter is here. It is 13:11.

This story shows my inner monologue through the embodiment process, as I found myself putting on and taking off that locket over and over again. I just knew that if I kept putting it back on I would find a sense of empowerment, and I did!

As experienced by Lauren Mahana

Pleasure in the Present

We mentioned earlier that an embodied birth produces oxytocin, which in turn creates love and also pleasure. Oxytocin is the magical hormone that helps our brains interpret birth as a pleasurable experience. This doesn't mean that every second of the birth is pleasurable— walking through the gates can often feel more painful than pleasurable—but the overall experience of birth can be one of pleasure, delight, empowerment, and love. We will speak extensively in Chapters 5 and 6 about creating a sacred space where pleasure can be most available to a laboring woman, but at the end of the day, our pleasure is ultimately our own responsibility. And the level of pleasure we experience, not just in birth but in life too, is directly related to how willing we are to being embodied and—how willing we are to be 100 percent in this now, present-moment—not the past, not the future, but here and now.

Being present sounds like an esoteric or Eastern religious teaching, but it is simpler than that. Being "present" means being aware, centered, grounded, and open to what is happening right now. When we are fully aware, we can't help but be fully embodied. So, awareness is another trick of the trade to walking through this gate as we saw in Lauren's birth story above. A huge benefit of being present is that it is really hard to experience fear (which lives in the past) and anxiety (which lives in the future)—two very prevalent emotions at most births. So just by being in the present and aware of the moment, we can eliminate two potentially destructive states of being for our oxytocin levels, meaning we have a greater opportunity to experience greater pleasure, and less pain, in our births simply by being present.

This state of being may be harder to invoke at the moment because we are not in the habit of practicing it consciously. We do, however, do it unconsciously all the time. Imagine a steamy and exciting sexual experience with a partner. Our minds, bodies, and spirits come fully into the present moment without effort. Our simple awareness and sensuality bring us into the present. We aren't thinking about what happened yesterday or the email we have to send later. No way! We are thinking about touch, taste, smell—our senses and pleasure. In fact, if we do start to think about our to-do list, it's usually an indication of a disconnect, and we notice that when our minds wander out of the present moment, we are no longer experiencing pleasure.

The same can be said of pregnancy, birth, and even postpartum. It's so tempting to allow ourselves to drift into the past or the future with fear and worry, but doing so risks losing all the pleasure that is available to us right now at this moment. If we can learn to harness embodiment through the simple practice of staying present and aware, we can instantly amplify our pleasure, our happiness, our satisfaction, and our feelings of connection with others. Depression and anxiety are typical symptoms of disembodiment because it is literally impossible for most people to be depressed or anxious when they are present. So how can we stay present? How can we learn to be embodied? The Integration Practices at the end of this chapter offer some solutions.

Empowered Birth is Self-Acceptance

We mentioned earlier that we commonly leave our bodies as a coping mechanism to avoid pain or discomfort—whether it's physical, emotional, or spiritual. But it is not just pain that we avoid. Sometimes we want to avoid some other part of ourselves. Usually, a part we dislike, feel shame around, or want to pretend doesn't exist. Denial is a powerful reason to disembody. But when we avoid our own truth, especially in labor, we abandon ourselves right when we need to be present the most. This is the time we need empowerment, and we need to be present to choose to walk through the Gates of Transformation.

But we can't do this if we resist our own self-acceptance. This gate is asking us to really look at and accept all parts of ourselves, and in doing so, we give our babies a great foundation for their own self-acceptance. But we have to choose it.

This is why the Maiden Goddess is given a choice to wear the locket or not. She can choose to learn to accept herself fully and face the good, the bad and the ugly and in doing so, finds self-acceptance and empowerment. Or she can choose to run away or hide, and in essence, abandon the opportunity to grow. It is very tempting to abandon ourselves, to disassociate and disconnect from our thoughts, feelings, memories, or sense of identity when pain, discomfort, awkwardness, and emotion show up in labor. But should we choose to embrace our truths and embrace the bad, we deepen our presence, deepen our embodiment and give our babies powerful energy to be born into. It's up to us. What will we choose?

In our experience as doulas, we've found that it is this embodiment piece that makes the difference between an empowered birth experience and a traumatic one—no matter what the actual circumstances are. What matters is how embodied mom was with each decision, each contraction, and each push that affects her level of personal satisfaction. And embodiment can only happen when fierce self-acceptance is observed.

The Cascade of Emotional Resistance to Embodiment

We talk a lot in the birth community about the idea of a "cascade of medical interventions" that can occur in hospital births. This is the idea that one medical intervention in birth—like breaking the bag of waters, inducing labor or getting an epidural—has the tendency to lead to another medical intervention and another until everything spins out of control and far from a natural, non-medicated birth experience. We've seen this cascade unfold more times than not. But what no one really talks about is what we call the "cascade of emotional resistance" that happens when we choose to or simply are unable to embody during labor due to trauma or medical reasons.

From our work as doulas, it's become clear to us that when women resist a gate, they run the risk of getting stuck there, and then have a higher chance of getting stuck at other gates. When they are stuck and not in their bodies, they sometimes end up making medical decisions from a place of "stuckness" or "autopilot" rather than from intention and purpose. This can lead to unwanted interventions or energies that are out of alignment with their Energetic Birth Plan (see Chapter 4).

Here's an example: let's say a mother wants her child birthed without medication finds that she is unable to walk through the Gate of Vulnerability mid-labor. Old shame around not being "good enough" shows up. She gets stuck at the gate and can't cope. So instead, she disembodies and numbs the experience through denial. Because she isn't in her body, she starts to feel victimized by labor and what the nurses are telling her. She starts to blame others as a way to soothe her emotional pain. She finds herself experiencing even deeper shame and pain as her baby descends down her birth canal.

Blaming others no longer is working, and she just can't walk through her gates, which causes even more pain. Shame is spiraling, and pain is increasing. The energy of her birth room shifts out of love and into fear and panic, increasing the risk of complications, her emotional suffering, and avoidance of her own power to transform. To ease her suffering, she asks for an epidural to find some kind of relief. She immediately feels grateful for the epidural's numbing effect on her physical pain, but she is now experiencing more shame than ever and feels a sense of dread, like she abandoned herself. Again, instead of coming back into her body now that the physical pain has subsided and facing the gates, she blames herself for not "being strong enough" to have the birth she wanted and stays stuck.

In her postpartum period, she continues to struggle with pain and feels victimized through her adventures with breastfeeding. It isn't until she goes to therapy that she starts to understand how her unprocessed shame set in motion a cascade of events that produced even more shame and more blame. With a therapist, she learns how to intentionally embody herself, forgive herself, and finally walk through the gates she resisted in labor. In doing so, she completes her transition into motherhood.

The "cascade of emotional resistance" in the explanation above is something that often happens when we are disembodied, running on autopilot and avoiding pain. A scenario like this is completely avoidable by simply being and practicing embodiment. It's clear that resisting emotional experiences, like shame, can ultimately affect our physical experience of birth. If you get one thing out of this chapter, let it be this: when we resist, we disembody; and when we disembody, we disempower ourselves. Being aware of your own habits and cascades of emotional resistance can help you tremendously when you arrive at labor, and the Integration Practices at the end of this chapter can help you prepare for it.

A DOULA'S BIRTH STORY

Laurel was a single mom who hired me to be her doula. She was only 24 years old and found herself unexpectedly pregnant. She had very little support from the father or family, so she was planning on having the baby on her own at the hospital with me. We talked about the gates only briefly because she insisted that she didn't need any emotional support since she had decided to get an epidural. I insisted we still talk about the gates, but I could only do so briefly. She resisted speaking about, or acknowledging, her feelings about her situation and used humor to move the conversation elsewhere. I could see she wasn't ready to face the emotional pain she was going through. So, we planned for an epidural, and I was just to be her physical support with massage, cool head towels, and push coaching.

When the day came, Laurel was surprised by the intensity of her contractions. We focused on breathing and moving. She was overwhelmed by the pain, and I encouraged her to share her feelings, but she resisted. When we arrived at the hospital, she asked for an epidural immediately and continued to labor. I kept encouraging her to talk to me and release whatever pent-up emotions there were, but she insisted on just focusing on getting through the physical contractions until the anesthesiologist arrived.

When he did, and the epidural was placed, it didn't work. Laurel felt numbness in her toes, but nowhere else. The medical staff repositioned the epidural, but Laurel still didn't experience any pain relief—it wasn't working. She was one of the small percentages of people who don't respond. This was when Laurel went into full panic mode. She had been relying on an epidural to keep her out of her body and out of her emotional pain, and without the epidural, she was brought to her knees. She was forced to be embodied in the experience, and I could see her becoming traumatized by it all. I started to talk to her about the locket and the power of embodiment. As we moved through each surge, I encouraged her to face her emotions which ended up being mostly shame for getting pregnant in the first place and loneliness for not reaching out to her family and trying to do it all on her own. It took her some time to face her gates, but she did, and with so much courage. I could see her powerfully transforming into a mother with each contraction and each surrender. It still makes me cry, thinking about her courage. When her baby finally arrived, I could see the transformation on her face. She did it—she faced the things she had resisted for nine months, and pure ecstatic joy emanated from her and from all who witnessed. The nurses couldn't stop remarking how powerful and brave she was—they were changed too. Laurel will forever be a reminder of the power of embodiment and how quickly we can move through the Gates of Transformation when we finally surrender to our own embodied experience.

As witnessed by Alexandria Moran

How to Walk Through the Gate of Embodiment

First, we must be willing to walk through all the gates as they show up. Next, we have to be willing to wear our lockets of embodiment. If we have any resistance to the gates, or to feeling all the feels, we are probably going to pop out of our bodies. This is okay if we recognize it and return as soon as we do. This is the dance of labor—facing a Gate of Transformation, resisting it, popping out of our bodies, deciding to return, surrendering to the sacrifice and finally finding the power in the surrender by crossing the threshold. This is what the Maiden Goddess does each time. But as doulas, we have a few tricks of the trade to share which we hope make embodiment just a little easier for you.

Embrace Sensuality

Sensuality is all about indulging and fulfilling the five senses: taste, touch, hearing, vision, and smell. When we focus on any one of our five senses, we automatically bring ourselves into the present moment, thereby bringing ourselves into our bodies. It is literally impossible to smell a rose and worry about the future at the same time. That is because our brain processes millions of bits of data all the time, yet makes sensory information a priority. So, whenever we indulge in a sense, our brain can't help but become present to the experience.

We learned earlier that being present provides the opportunity for embodiment, which comes from pleasure. So if we don't just smell the rose, but invoke pleasure from it, we have immediately created a space where we are present and embodied. As doulas, this is an amazing trick to use in labor, and when we see a mom resisting a gate and looking to avoid, numb, or run away, we offer her a scent or a taste or a beautiful image, and she immediately returns to herself and can face the gate with empowerment. Describing your personal preferences for sensual experiences can be a great addition to your Energetic Birth Plan (see Chapter 4) and can help your birth partner get you back into your body when you pop out.

The other benefit of sensuality is that it focuses our attention on something pleasurable—like a piece of dark chocolate melting in the mouth—and away from a painful sense—like the contracting uterus. The brain can only process one thing at a time, and pleasure tends to win when we allow it. So, if we give ourselves pleasurable and sensual experiences in labor, not only can we minimize painful sensation, but we also increase oxytocin (the natural epidural) which makes labor much more manageable. And when we are in pleasure, we want to stay in pleasure, which makes it so much easier to stay embodied.

Free Your Sexuality

There is a strong unspoken taboo in our culture that birth isn't sexual, nor should it be. We also have the same judgment on motherhood: that a mother should be a Madonna and have no sexual desire or appeal.

The patriarchy (the underlying and often subconscious system in our culture that values masculinity over femininity) can't accept the fact that birth is inherently sexual, and mothers are too. Because we are influenced by the world we live in, as women, we've disconnected our sexuality from our experience of birth and motherhood to abide by the cultural norms. But this truly does us a disservice not only in terms of our embodiment but also in terms of our sexual sovereignty. Why should an experience that revolves around our sexual organs not be sexual? Are we so disconnected from ourselves that we would rather have a painful birth than a sexual one? The collective would say yes, but as birth workers, we want to shout "Hell no!"

The idea of an orgasmic birth seems so far out of left field for many of us that we don't even consider it a possibility. But the truth is, when you are embodied, you have access to a whole world of experiences that are otherwise out of reach. And one of the most effective ways of becoming embodied is through sexual activation. If you are willing to be sexual throughout labor, you have more opportunities to be embodied and experience pleasure. But you have to give yourself permission first and face any personal and collective shame.

It's also a great idea to set aside time for some connection with your partner/husband/wife/girlfriend/boyfriend during labor. Making these sexy moments of intimacy and connection a priority has been proven to reduce pain, which always helps with embodiment. If privacy is an issue, and you don't want to go the full monty, these intimate moments can be done in the bathroom or behind a closed door as described below. Achieving a sense of safety is key to feeling that full pleasure embodiment. After all, you probably had privacy to become sexual and make the baby. You may want to recreate that atmosphere when you labor. We often encourage this in labor and have found that moms who engage in sexual expression tend to feel the happiest about their birth experiences. Sexy births = oxytocin births.

Create Privacy

Birth tends to be an experience where there are many witnesses (nurses, birth partners, family members, doctors), so we are very aware of the fact that as we labor, we are being watched. This can sometimes be a block to our embodiment because we are afraid of looking a certain way. Because let's face it, pleasure in our society is something that happens behind closed doors. Could you imagine being in a restaurant as a woman orgasmically indulges in cheesecake? Moaning as she twirls the spoon around her tongue in delight? Most people would feel mortified, even though she is not doing anything sexual, except eating with pleasure. That is because we are still uncomfortable with women enjoying pleasure in our society. So now imagine a pleasurable birth experience. All that shame comes into the birth space.

As doulas, we often create as much privacy as possible for the laboring mom to reduce levels of shame or judgment projected from bystanders. This way, mom can labor in pleasure as she pleases without the gavel of modesty ready to come smashing down. Closing doors, curtains, and windows while dimming lights can be great non-verbal cues to onlookers that this is a private experience. Another great doula trick to get privacy is just getting naked. You'll see how fast a room clears out when there is a naked woman laboring in her full glory. No one will come until you ask for them.

A DOULA'S BIRTH STORY

Megan and Dave were the cutest couple. They were very affectionate with each other at our prenatal appointments, and I could tell there was a lot of love between them. I was so excited to be their doula because I knew that the sexy energy between partners at birth always makes for the most embodied and easy experiences for mamas. I often teach my couples to be touchy with each other throughout pregnancy, but Megan and Dave just had so much natural affection. They wanted to have an all-natural birth and soaked up all the information I could give them on the Gates of Transformation. It was clear that they were a power couple and had deep emotional intimacy.

When the day came, they called me only when they were on their way to the hospital because they had been coping so well—just the two of them at home with massage, kisses, and love. When we arrived at the hospital, Megan was dilated 8 cm and smiling through her contractions as Dave kissed her neck and rubbed her back. They arrived too late to be offered an epidural, which was their plan all along. Because she was so embodied, the disappointment of not having her birth plan go the way she wanted didn't even faze her. They continued to labor together and asked me several times to step out of the room so they could have some intimacy. Within two hours, Megan was pushing out her baby and kissing Dave in between each push, and he kept whispering words of affirmation and love in her ear. It took only three pushes, and she was holding her baby in her arms. Her total labor was a short seven hours total from start to finish. The nurses and doctors were surprised, but I knew it was all the oxytocin they had produced with their affectionate connection and trust. This was truly a sexy birth.

As witnessed by Alexandria Moran

Move the Body

Another doula trick of the trade to get embodied is through movement. Physically move your body by dancing, walking, shaking, and swaying. Get the blood pumping through your body. When we focus on physical movements, and especially movements that feel good and invoke pleasure, our souls can't help but re-embody. This is why movement is one of the top comfort measures taught in childbirth preparation. Movement has the power to embody instantaneously because it engages multiple senses, and it also because it releases endorphins and other precursors to oxytocin that make us feel good.

As doulas, we often encourage our laboring moms to dance and allow the pleasure of the music to unfold within their bodies. Getting lost in the present experience is a great way to know that we've embodied ourselves. Just like with sexuality and sensuality, this can sometimes require a level of privacy to fully embrace the process. If you don't surrender to the music but rather try to perform for those that may be watching, you aren't actually embodying so this may also be something that can be done behind closed doors.

Sometimes in birth, movement is limited as in the case of an epidural when moms are bedridden and physically numb. Being disconnected from any physical sensations and movement can make it easier to disembody, which is why we believe movement is most important for bedridden moms.

Just because you can't move your legs doesn't mean you can't focus your attention on other forms of movement or sensation. Stretch your upper body, focus on your breath, or get your birth partner to massage your shoulders or hands. Bring any other form of physical pleasure, sensory attention, or movement back to the body (see Appendix IV *Doula Tips to Have an Empowered Epidural Birth*). Whenever the body is in pleasure, the spirit wants to join in, so creating as many experiences of pleasure as possible is a sure way to be embodied throughout labor, even if you can't move too much.

INTEGRATION PRACTICES

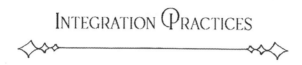

The following practices are intended to help you integrate the information of this chapter and apply it to your life now, so you can walk through this gate with embodiment and mindfulness while in labor. Take your time going through the practices that resonate the most with you and feel free to do them as often as you'd like.

SELF-LOVE ACTIVITY: BEING PRESENT THROUGH GROUNDING

Learning to ground is one of the most powerful ways to embody with intention. It is as simple as imagining a golden rope extending from your womb all the way down into the center of the Earth, wrapping around its core and anchoring your body and soul to the planet. Practicing this visualization daily can be very helpful in practicing embodiment. Visit www.laborlikeagoddess.com to download one of our many grounding meditations.

Other ways to ground yourself are to walk barefoot on the earth, grass, or dirt to squat over the earth. This allows the energy of the earth to connect with your own energy and can bring a very grounded sense to the body and soul. Earthy scents like pine and cedar also have a very powerful grounding effect and can be used in labor. Smelling these before labor starts can be a powerful way to practice embodiment.

Finally, mantras, affirmations, and meditations all help with grounding as they give the mind something to do and bring you into the present moment, so embodiment is more available. Visit www.laborlikeagoddess. com for grounding offerings.

SELF-LOVE ACTIVITY: RAISING OXYTOCIN

As mentioned earlier in the chapter, the more oxytocin you produce during labor, the more love, embodiment, and pleasure will be available to you. But you don't have to wait for labor to start to increase your oxytocin bank account. You can start adding to it now in pregnancy through daily acts of pleasure. Commit to doing one thing daily that brings a sense of peace and pleasure to your life. It can be anything that raises your oxytocin levels and brings love into your space. Some examples: put clean, new sheets on your bed, diffuse your favorite essential oil, get a massage, make your favorite dessert, go for a walk in nature, get your nails done, buy a new outfit, pleasure yourself, sing in the shower, or kiss your lover.

SELF-LOVE ACTIVITY: LOCKET OF EMBODIMENT

Give yourself a physical reminder of the sacrifice of this gate—buy a locket or create a talisman pouch that you can wear around your neck to inspire embodiment. If you get a locket, you might like to place an image or item inside that is meaningful to you. Some mamas will put a mini image of their ultrasound photo in it. If you want to create a talisman pouch, you can collect a few different items that are special to you and help you remain embodied, such as special crystals, feathers, or jewelry. You can wear this throughout pregnancy and labor as a sacred tool or reminder and motivation to practice embodiment.

INNER EXPLORATION JOURNAL PROMPTS

The following journal prompts are for you to explore and uncover the different challenges of this gate. The practice of journaling can be deeply healing and enlightening, so we encourage you to spend some time reading over the prompts to see which ones resonate with you. Look back at these often. You might notice that different journal prompts resonate at different times. We also recommend doing these journal entries after practicing some grounding to help process and bring to light deeper truths and understandings.

Embodiment

- When do I feel the most embodied in my life?
- When do I numb myself, disassociate, or avoid?
- What activities make me leave my body (e.g.,TV, drugs, shopping, social media)?
- What activities make me return to my body (e.g., pleasure, massage, sex, food)?
- What gates do I usually resist? What gates are hard for me?
- Does my resistance cause a cascade of emotions and experiences? If so, what are they?
- How can I bring more embodiment to my pregnancy, labor, and postpartum experience?
- How does it feel when I'm not embodied? How does it feel when I am?
- When do I abandon myself?
- How can I show up for myself and my baby when I want to disembody?

Sensuality

- How often do I invoke sensuality in my life?
- What areas of my life would I like to add more sensuality?
- How does being sensual make me feel?
- Do I prefer a certain sense/senses? If so, which one(s)?
- Do I neglect a certain sense/senses? If so, which one(s)?

Sexuality

- How comfortable am I with my own sexuality?
- How comfortable am I with my sexuality being expressed in birth?
- What makes me feel safe when I have sex? Can I bring that sense to my birth space?

- Do I want to be sexual with my life partner in labor? Why or why not?
- If not, can I find sexuality with myself in labor? Why or why not?
- How do I feel about self-pleasuring in labor?
- What fears do I have around my sexuality? What shames? Can I face these before labor?
- When do I feel the sexiest?
- When do I feel the most confidence?
- When do I stop myself from experiencing pleasure?

GODDESS RITUAL: FACING THE GOOD, THE BAD, AND THE UGLY

Do this ritual on a New Moon as a way of connecting and embracing all aspects of yourself. Becoming comfortable with your own body, emotions, thought processes, and patterns can be really difficult, hence the need to escape from yourself. But when we abandon ourselves, we lose our power. This ritual is meant to help you reclaim your inner power by visually looking at the good, the bad, and the ugly aspects of ourselves.

What You Need:

- A piece of paper
- A pen
- A lighter
- A fireproof bowl
- A New Moon

What to Do:

Under the New Moon, fold a piece of paper in thirds, lengthwise, to create three columns. At the top of each column, label them "Good," "Bad," and "Ugly." Spend a few minutes grounding either by walking barefoot on the earth or using a grounding meditation. When you are ready, start to list in each column, the things you consider about yourself to be "good," to be "bad," and to be "ugly" — in other words, things you like, things you don't like and you'd rather deny about yourself. When the lists are complete, read and observe your lists. Ask yourself if you're ready to face the good, the bad, and the ugly. Are you ready to stop running and fully accept the truth of who you are right now? Notice if there is any resistance. If so, do some more grounding. But if you are ready to fully embrace your truth, light the paper on fire. Allow the fire to transmute and shift the energy of resistance into the energy of acceptance. Try to imagine the smoke dissolving it in your body. Allow the paper to burn all the way down.

Bury the ashes in the dirt and know that you are ready to fully walk through this gate when it shows up. Feel free to do this as many times as you need for as many New Moons are necessary. Only you will know when it feels complete.

GODDESS RITUAL: MAIDEN-TO-MOTHER AFFIRMATION

Say the following affirmation as often as you like aloud, quietly or as a mantra over and over again as you transition from Maiden-to-Mother. Place your hands over your heart chakra and say: *"I embrace all experiences that are on my path, I am truly present and embodied!"*

THRESHOLD MEDITATION

Threshold meditations are meant to help you cross a gate when you are ready. In this meditation, you'll go on a short journey through this gate, while wearing a metaphorical locket so you can choose to embody your entire experience of pregnancy and labor. This is a perfect meditation if you tend to numb, distract, avoid, abandon, or deny your pain, discomfort, shame, or fear. This practice can be done after each journal prompt or daily until you feel complete in your transition. It is also a great meditation for labor when those popping-out-of-body moments really hit. Visit www.laborlikeagoddess.com to download it.

Final Thoughts

Throughout this chapter, we have discussed how becoming embodied allows us to fully commit to being an active participant in labor and allows us to experience the greatest amount of joy, pleasure, and satisfaction with our birth experience. Hopefully, you now truly understand what embodiment means for you and how you can practice embodiment in your daily life. Wearing the Locket of Embodiment is hard work at first, and it does require a level of personal accountability and awareness to put in the time for self-work. We promise that if you spend some time with the Integration Practices and start to get comfortable with becoming embodied on demand, you will soar through this gate in labor. The hardest step is just believing in yourself, so just know that we believe in you!

~ CHAPTER VI ~

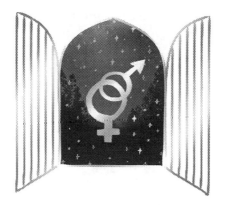

THE GATE OF SACRED PARTNERSHIP

OPENING TO THE DIVINE MASCULINE

You have half our gifts. I the other. Together we make a whole. Together we are much more powerful.

—*Joss Stirling*

The Maiden Goddess continued her journey feeling expansive, yet also feeling the effects of all the gates she had passed through. It was as if everything in her experience had been turned up 10,000 percent. The pain, the shame the fear, the anxiety—everything she avoided, she had to feel, which was a new sensation for her. An exhausting one.

The Maiden Goddess found herself slowing down under the heavy weight of the locket. Her muscles ached, the cold that hadn't bothered her before now started to give her chills, and she began to shut down. So much so, that she eventually stopped walking from the utter exhaustion of embodiment and collapsed on the ground. Her body wasn't used to it. Her ego wasn't used to it. And soon she was unable to move one more inch.

She thought, "There is no way I can continue, and there is no way I can sleep. There is no shelter; I will freeze if I don't keep moving, but I just can't move anymore." She was starting to doze off when a fifth gate appeared, just like the four before, big, iron-clad, and enchanted. The Maiden Goddess was so tired she could barely knock, but she did, and a fifth crone appeared asking what business she had knocking on her door.

"I long to become a mother. I wish to go to the Underworld," the Maiden Goddess barely could communicate. She thought, "I am a joke. How can I possibly continue to the Underworld in such a state?" She longed for a break, for a good night's rest, for a chance to recover.

"Ah yes, I see," said the Gatekeeper, "Then you will have to walk through this gate, but I will only let you pass if you give me your ability to walk."

"Huh?" The Maiden Goddess couldn't tell if she was confused or if this Gatekeeper was messing with her. "How can I walk across this gate if I can't walk? That's absurd!"

But the Gatekeeper only replied, "That is the sacrifice required. You will just need to learn how to call upon and rely on the help of others."

"Others? What others?" The Maiden Goddess thought to herself. She looked around, and there was clearly no one else for miles. But her thoughts drifted to her beloved. Oh, how she missed him and longed for his support. He would surely help her walk through this threshold, maybe even carry her.

She dreamed about him for a while. When she opened her eyes, she couldn't believe it, but he was standing right in front of her, his hand reaching down toward her. Was she hallucinating from the exhaustion? Was it him? Or was this the Gatekeeper's cruel joke?

It was him. The Maiden Goddess summoned him, and he appeared, willing and able to help her.

She was incredibly grateful and yet, found herself feeling deeply embarrassed by the state of herself. What a fright she must have seemed to him, she thought. And she felt like a complete failure that she couldn't complete this journey on her own and needed his help.

She knew she needed to ask for his help but couldn't quite bring herself to. She felt her independence and sense of self slipping away. But when she looked into her beloved's eyes, she felt his deep love and admiration for her, and it softened her heart. She said to herself, "There is strength and power in asking for help, and I will not allow my ego to keep me suffering. I open my heart to others and receive the help that is so willingly offered to me with deep reverence and gratitude."

So she asked for his help and opened herself up to his strength and support. The gates flung open and he effortlessly picked her up and the two of them, together, crossed the threshold.

She was overcome with such gratitude for his loving support and the opportunity to rest in his arms. She slept and recovered as he carried her through to the next gate. She couldn't expect that she would need every last ounce of energy for what lay ahead.

The Importance of Birth Partners

An empowered birth is one that is supported by at least one birth partner whose main focus is to promote, validate, and honor our emotional, spiritual, and physical transition into motherhood during labor. The birth partner is someone who can empower us, help us reclaim our strength, and encourage us to trust ourselves more deeply as we surrender into the unknown Underworld of labor. This is a special relationship that provides the necessary support when the thought of moving through a Gate of Transformation becomes too much to handle on our own. As doulas, it is our job to fulfill the role of the birth partner. But birth partners can also be the baby's father, or grandmother, a family friend, a sister, or a nurse—anyone who can witness, support, and encourage a laboring mother to have an empowered birth experience.

The number one job of any birth partner is to create an environment where we can fully immerse ourselves in our birthing energy and flow, so that the wild woman within, the one who instinctively knows how to bring a baby into the world, can emerge with full power. Without proper support, it can be really difficult for this primal aspect of ourselves to show up. Because let's face it, we spend most of our lives trying to suppress this wild woman so we can be deemed "respectable." So when she shows up in birth—and she always does—we're going to want a friendly face to cheer us on when every part of ourselves wants to run away and hide to maintain whatever sense of dignity we can, so we don't have to feel embarrassed by the shameless, savage energy that will inevitably emerge.

Without this supportive environment, we run the risk of getting stuck in our analytical brains (the masculine side of ourselves) and turning off our natural instincts to labor (the feminine side of ourselves). When we disconnect from these natural instincts, all kinds of complications can show up that require medical interventions and sometimes even emergency surgery. However, if we prepare with a good birth partner and have the privacy, time, space, and permission to invoke that instinctual feminine nature with a partner who is right there by our side, we can labor and birth with much fewer complications. Because the natural energy of birth is feminine surrender: surrender to the gates, surrender to the body, surrender to the baby, surrender to the spiritual death—feminine surrender.

It is important to understand that doctors and nurses are responsible for the physical wellbeing and safety of mom and baby. We can't really look to them for emotional support. It is not in their job description, and unless they are especially compassionate, they are not usually thinking about the emotional or psychological ramifications of their actions. So having a doula or birth partner whose main focus is to support the emotional, physical, and spiritual transformation of birth will round out the birth experience and offer a more holistically supportive experience. Many women in hindsight wish they had spent the time and effort building their birth team and creating this level of support for themselves. We've never heard a woman wish she didn't have emotional or spiritual support.

Birth is a Divine Feminine Expression

Within each of us are masculine and feminine sides to our personalities, Yin and yang, no matter what gender we identify with. Depending on how we were raised and what culture we grew up in, we each have a natural inclination toward one energy or the other. Since the worldwide feminist movement, women have learned to embrace more of their masculinity as a means of surviving and thriving in a male-dominated society. To succeed in a career, it is much more valuable to display attributes that are more masculine than feminine. For example, at work it is more helpful to be direct, linear, straightforward, action-oriented, and unemotional (all masculine qualities) than it is to be dreamy, intuitive, internally focused, or cyclical (all feminine qualities). So, we learned how to harness the masculine side of ourselves to succeed at work.

If you don't believe us, just ask yourself: when was the last time you told your boss that you couldn't come in because you were bleeding and the Moon was asking you to journal instead? Probably never, because feminine qualities at work are not praised, they can be grounds for dismissal. And although that seems like an outlandish scenario, it really displays the difference between the masculine and feminine energies in our world and the value we place on each of them. Both are useful for certain experiences. Our masculine energy is incredibly useful in our careers and providing for ourselves and for our families financially. But labor and birth are where our feminine qualities shine, and it is beneficial to let our masculine energy sit on the sidelines when the baby wants to be born.

This is because birth is all about embracing and embodying the energy of our inner Divine Feminine. When we do so, we learn to spiral within our emotions, cycle through our surges, go within, connect to our own transformation and allow our minds to drift into a dreamy trance of birth fog. However, if our masculine side shows up in birth, with its to-do's, its action-oriented checklists, and its continuous scanning for danger, it disrupts the feminine trusting energy we need to be fully immersed in labor. Instead, we start to use our analytical mind, rather than our intuitive mind, or look at labor as a linear journey—checking off each gate as a destination, rather than a spiraling swirl of contraction and expansion. Just like it's better to keep our feminine side at bay at work, it is better to keep our masculine side at bay in birth.

Knowing the Difference Between Our Masculine and Feminine Sides

But to do so, we have to be able to recognize within ourselves when our masculine side shows up and when our feminine side shows up. Just ask yourself, when was the last time you let your feminine energy call the shots in your day? When was the last time you let yourself daydream, journal, dance, meditate, and go-within, all without an agenda, timeline, or linear structure? Maybe never? Maybe yesterday? This answer will help us understand just how underdeveloped your feminine side actually is.

If you have an underdeveloped feminine side, it is very important to do the Integration Practices at the end of this chapter to help you embrace your feminine self and unpack the things that make you uncomfortable about the feminine. Vulnerability is a big reason most women don't want to even touch their feminine side. It often makes us feel too exposed, and we have a history that tells us that needing others ends in disappointment, unmet needs, a feeling of helplessness, victimization, and in extreme cases, betrayal. If this is the case, we suggest going through the Gate of Vulnerability as much as you can to start to break down this barrier and accept vulnerability as a quality of strength, rather than a weakness as many of us have been taught to believe.

Accepting Help from Others

Birth is all about vulnerability, and one of the biggest acts of vulnerability is being able to ask for help from others and receive that help with a gracious heart. We often find this very difficult to do as our masculine-style upbringings usually teach us, either directly or subliminally, that asking for help shows weakness, which is unacceptable in our society. So, instead, we learn to hide any sense of vulnerability and try to do everything on our own, even at the risk of harming our own emotional or mental stability. This false sense of independence is responsible for so much burnout, anger and unknown resentment in women, impatience in mothers, and low-level anxiety and/or depression.

In our story, the sacrifice the Maiden Goddess must give is her ability to walk. Her mobility is what grants her the greatest independence in her mind; it's what will allow her to achieve her dream of motherhood on her own. But the Gatekeeper knows that she cannot become a mother on her own. Motherhood requires the ego to relax and ask for support, even when it feels vulnerable, or rather *because* it feels vulnerable. This is how the Maiden can start to move out of her goal-oriented masculine energy and into her receptive and expansive feminine energy.

We've mentioned before that we used to live in communities that had built-in support for new mothers. There was always someone to hand the baby to so we could take a shower, or just have an hour to lie on the grass to recharge. But in our independence-obsessed culture, moms today are saddled with our babies 24/7 without relief or support or sometimes even just a moment to use the bathroom. It's overwhelming, stressful, and doesn't create happy families.

Mothers need support. Period. We need it once the baby is here AND when we are laboring. We need it so we can be fully in our Divine Feminine energy, and we can use our support system to hold the energy of the Divine Masculine, so we don't have to. Since it isn't built into our society like it used to be, as mothers, we have to seek out and create this kind of support for ourselves. *We have to ask.* We have to create it so we can allow ourselves to be carried by our support system, giving us full permission to leave our own inner masculine on the sideline, because our support system is holding that energy.

This is especially important in labor. We must be fully in our feminine energies, which means we need to create a support system or partnership that can hold the energy of the Divine Masculine on our behalf, so we don't have to. Because it is only when we feel safe in the Divine Masculine energy will we be able to let our own inner masculine take a break. We are safe, protected, and honored as we allow ourselves to be fully immersed in our Wild Woman feminine archetype.

The Two Forces of Creation

We've touched on how each of us has an internal masculine and feminine side to ourselves. Creation does too—it is a requirement. It takes the Divine Feminine (an egg) and the Divine Masculine (a sperm) to conceive a new life. Two opposing forces had to join in a beautiful and miraculous union to *create*.

The same energy it takes to make a baby is the same energy required to birth a baby into the world. Labor requires the Divine Feminine surrendering into the Divine Masculine for a sacred energetic union to occur. To birth easily, efficiently, and peacefully, we must be able to fully embody our Divine Feminine self so we can be fully open to the energy of trust, sacrifice, and intuitive spiraling. But we can only do that if there is an opposing force keeping the space safe for this deep vulnerability. We must have the Divine Masculine force holding the space and guarding the energy for the Divine Feminine to express. This can be a husband, a birth partner, a father, a sister, a mother, a nurse, a doctor, or a friend.

The presence of the Divine Masculine is a crucial element of any birth and one that is not really understood and is often neglected. The most empowered births are births that are supported with the steady, strong, protective, and fierce energy of the Divine Masculine. These are the births that tend to be the most magical, peaceful, and pleasurable.

Because we all have Divine Feminine and Divine Masculine energy within us, anyone can hold the space of the Divine Masculine no matter their gender preference. So, a cisgender man isn't the only one who can hold this space. We've seen beautiful all-female birth teams that are shining examples of the Divine Masculine. We've also seen gay brothers, uncles, grandpas, doulas, nurses, and doctors all hold the Divine Masculine space. It doesn't matter *who* is holding the space, just that *someone* is. What is important is that there is at least one person whose sole job it is to hold the space sacred for the birthing mother and child. When we have this sacred birth partner, birth can be an incredibly supportive, pleasurable, and fulfilling experience. It makes it so much easier to go through each gate because we are held in divine energy.

On our website, we've created two e-books specifically to help your birth team truly understand how to do this for you. The first is called *Help A Women Labor Like A Goddess: A How-To Manual for the Birth Partner*. The second eBook is called *Become the God So Your Woman Can Labor Like A Goddess*. Each book goes into detail on how to be the Divine Masculine energy at the birth of your baby. Visit www.laborlikeagoddess.com to download them.

Understanding the Divine Masculine Energy

The Divine Masculine is the energy on our planet that embodies strength, protection, support, action, compassion, heroism, confidence, power, discernment, and unconditional love. Think about the characters of King Arthur, Santa or Mufasa. They each embody what it means to be in the Divine Masculine energy. There is a sense of safety, leadership, and comfort when we are in their presence. Being grounded is soothing when we feel lost or out of control. As laboring women, this energy gives us the sense that *everything is okay no matter what happens,* which gives us permission to do what we need to do in labor. We don't have to be on the lookout for danger because we trust and know that someone else is.

The Divine Masculine energy makes the birthplace feel safe, protected, and in peace. Its main concern is keeping the room calm, peaceful, quiet, dark, and private at all times. When the energy of mom starts to turn to fear, anxiety, anger, or frustration, the Divine Masculine offers soft, reassuring eyes, and strong arms to hold her as she moves through her gates.

Just like in our story, the Divine Masculine is a breath of fresh air for the laboring woman. It's the steady oak tree she can lean on, and it won't sway no matter how messy, wounded, hurt, beat down, and emotional she may be. There is no judgment, no ridicule, no fear in the Divine Masculine, only utter love and admiration for the woman laboring and moving through her Gates of Ttransformation. This is what we all wish to have in our birth rooms so we can feel free to labor as we please, knowing we have strong arms to fall back on.

A DOULA'S BIRTH STORY

Keith supported his girlfriend Maya in the hospital in his full Divine Masculine energy. Since they hired a doula, they had talked about what she needed from him and created an Energetic Birth Plan together (see Chapter 4). It was understood that the best way Keith could support Maya was to keep the room calm and peaceful and do whatever needed to be done to keep labor progressing. Maya knew that she wanted the doula at her side at all times, so Keith would be the one to run errands and make sure the ambiance was peaceful so Maya could labor with the doula.

And that is exactly what he did. He kept the cup of ice chips full, the lights dim, asked for the machines to be turned to silent, pasted a "silence please" note on the door, kept the music pleasurable, made sure Maya had a mobile monitoring belt for baby's heartbeat and constantly checked in with how she was doing. He basically did all the behind the scenes work to make the room as peaceful, beautiful, and calm as was possible.

The nurse working with them respected the energy he was creating and came in as quietly as she could to avoid disrupting Maya's labor as little possible. And Maya was progressing steadily. But then there was a shift change with the nurses and the new nurse assigned to them didn't seem to have the same level of awareness. She would flip the lights on each time she came in, adjust the AC, speak very loudly, and be very disruptive in checking on mom. She did this several times, and Keith noticed that Maya was starting to experience more pain than she had been because she kept getting pulled out of her birth trance. After talking about it with Maya, they agreed that Keith would ask the nurse to be more conscious of the peaceful atmosphere that was important to the labor. He took the nurse aside, out of earshot of Maya, and explained what they wished. The nurse didn't react well, and so Keith said that she might not be the best fit, and that he would like to have another nurse assigned to them.

The nurse seemed relieved to be reassigned, and the new nurse who joined through the delivery respected the serene birth experience Keith was maintaining. Maya was very grateful and was very minimally disturbed all because Keith was able to hold the Divine Masculine energy of protection throughout the labor. Both Keith and Maya felt very empowered about the experience.

As witnessed by Alexandria Moran

Understanding the Wounded Masculine Energy

In contrast, the wounded masculine energy is the exact opposite of the Divine Masculine energy. If the Divine expresses love, the wounded expresses everything but love. It is this version of the masculine that we are perhaps more accustomed to in our society. It's what patriarchy stems from and more often than not, it can show up in the birth room and cause emotional and physical discomfort for the laboring woman. The wounded masculine embodies immaturity and is uncomfortable with the energy of transformation. He often doesn't know how to act so he will either stand on the sidelines, with his hands in his pockets or become controlling, cruel, or arrogant, inserting himself into the birth experience without invitation or awareness. He is less concerned about the laboring woman that his own insecurities and ego. Because we all have a masculine side, we've seen the wounded masculine show up in all kinds of people in the birth room, from female nurses, to doctors, to husbands, to even the laboring woman herself!

The wounded masculine is hurt, but because of his immaturity, he can't express it, so he lashes out or manipulates others to get what he wants. He makes the laboring woman feel like her labor is too [*fill in the blank*] long/intense/inconvenient/etc. The birth becomes about him and not about the baby's first expression in the world or the mother's brave journey into her Underworld.

It is the job of the Divine Masculine to keep any and all wounded masculine energy out of the birth space. That may mean kicking out in-laws or even firing nurses. The wounded masculine has a way of toxifying the birth experience for everyone involved, so it is so important that at least one person on our birth team is holding that Divine Masculine space.

A DOULA'S BIRTH STORY

This story is a little different than the rest. Most of my stories happen within the first few hours if not days of my clients' births, but not this story. Grant became a father about a year ago, and overall, the first year was okay. He would describe it as a year that was full of as many joys as struggles. He was really happy to be a father and that his daughter was happy and healthy, but something was missing. Grant struggled with the fact he didn't fall completely in love with his baby girl right away. He was ashamed. He never told his wife or anyone about his feelings, because he feared judgment or that he might be a bad dad. Over the past year, he had struggled with this notion that he loved his daughter, but he wasn't in love with her. Grant described it by saying, "I would die for her, I would give my life for hers, but when we are together, I don't feel that ooey-gooey love. I thought something was wrong with me."

Grant's wife Rachel exclusively breastfed, and they also co-slept with the baby. Grant felt a disconnect from his wife and child throughout this process. He wasn't included in the intimate moments of their daily life and felt like an outsider in his own family. Grant was too afraid to express his feelings to his wife, and he didn't know what to say. So, he pretended that everything was fine—until one day, about eight months postpartum, he got angry with his wife.

Grant screamed and shouted about how he wasn't a good father, and that he didn't know how to love. Rachel was shocked and surprised that this was how he felt.

After having a long conversation, Rachel and Grant realized that it wasn't that Grant didn't love his daughter. It was that he felt disconnected from her and from his wife. They came up with many ways to help Grant feel more included in the dynamic in the way he needed which included Rachel verbally inviting Grant to participate in daily life and also giving him more one-on-one time with Rachel so his own needs could be met. This made all the difference, and now Grant feels very fulfilled and in love with his little family.

As witnessed by Lauren Mahana

Resisting the Divine Masculine

We mentioned earlier that even laboring moms can display aspects of the wounded masculine by not letting their own masculine sit on the sidelines. When we do this, we end up being on full alert our entire labor and never fully emerging as Divine Feminine expression. This usually happens when we have trust issues or perhaps past trauma. When we allow our own wounded masculine to run the show, we are not surrendering to the Divine Masculine Energy in birth. If this resonates with you, we highly recommend spending extra time going through all the gates so you can allow yourself to truly be vulnerable in birth.

The other way we resist the Divine Masculine is by allowing our wounded feminine side to rule the show. This is usually displayed as the attitude that we can do it all in birth or we don't want to burden anyone with our needs. Women who take this attitude in labor often end up having a traumatic birth experience. That is why being able to move through this gate is crucial. And because we can't birth alone, there will be many times where we feel like we can't continue without surrendering to the Divine Masculine—which actually gives us renewed strength. We need the Divine Masculine to take us to the next gate many times throughout labor, we just need to be willing to be carried.

One of the biggest red flags of the wounded feminine is this resistance to being carried, supported, or helped by others. In our story, the Maiden Goddess has a moment where she isn't sure if she can surrender to the help being offered. She feels shame and disappointment for not being able to do it on her own. In labor, we too have these moments. But if we can surrender to the Divine Masculine, we will move through this gate.

We've often seen how resistance is the point of trauma. The Divine Masculine energy is there, but mom refuses to be supported by it. Instead, she insists on doing it on her own, and labor somehow becomes a bit harder and more painful for her. Often, when she looks back on the experience, she feels wronged and victimized by it. But the truth is, she just wouldn't let herself be carried, and this resistance prevented her from walking through this gate. So, we must start to practice asking for help now, in pregnancy, so it will be second nature during labor.

How to ~~Walk~~ Be Carried Through the Gate of Sacred Partnership

The previous gates required us to walk through on our own with our heads held high. This gate, however, is asking us to surrender to the help, support, and strength of others. We must learn to give up our independence—our desire to do everything solo—and look to the Divine Masculine for help. The Maiden Goddess literally must allow herself to be carried across the threshold by her Beloved. This can bring up all kinds of feelings of vulnerability, shame, fear, and stress that must be worked through to cross this gate effectively.

Set up a Sacred Partnership

The first thing we must do is set up a Sacred Partnership either with a doula, a friend, a family member, or the baby's dad. Make sure they understand what it means to be the Divine Masculine force in the labor room and are emotionally mature enough to hold that kind of space for you. Have them download our e-book so they can fully understand their role. Also, make sure they can be present for the entire experience from the beginning of labor all the way through a few hours after birth. This means they are "on-call" two weeks before the estimated due date and two weeks after. Talk with your partner about the divine energies you would like present at birth and what makes you feel safe when things get scary. Being able to communicate your needs to the Divine Masculine and give direct feedback is crucial in creating this Sacred Partnership.

When you are ready, it's a great idea to create a sacred contract between the two of you. Think of it as a vow for the birth day that also outlines roles, boundaries, safe words, and understandings between the two of you. The more personal you get, the more powerful this contract becomes. So dig deep. Check out Appendix II for an example of a Sacred Partnership Contract. This is the exact contract created between on of the authors, Alexandria Moran, and her husband. This is personal to their relationship and their needs. Yours can look completely different. Just make it personal. It is really important to do this ahead of time to ensure the most empowered and authentic experience. Discussing the contract before labor begins can help the entire birth team get on the same page. You can create multiple Sacred Partnerships or just one—whatever works for you. Just make sure you do it ahead of time. If you go into labor without establishing a Divine Masculine force, you may end up grasping at anything that remotely resembles the Divine Masculine and giving away your power to family members, doctors, doulas or any other person present. Whenever we give our power over and lose our sovereignty, disempowerment soon follows. So, make a Sacred Partnership something you do in advance.

Learn to Surrender to the Divine Masculine Energy

Once the day of labor arrives, you need to actually surrender to this Sacred Partnership—which is often easier said than done, unless you've been practicing your entire pregnancy, which we highly recommend. As with everything in this book, the more you practice ahead of time, the easier it is to do so on the big day. So have practice sessions with your Sacred Partner. Communicate your wants and needs, and let them know how to best support you when you feel vulnerable and scared.

Surrendering to the Divine Masculine is often much easier in theory than in practice, which is why we highly recommend doing the exercises in the book or working with a professional. If you have a history of trauma, disappointment, or violence with the masculine, this gate may be difficult to surrender to. Or if you are someone who prefers to do everything on your own and never asks for help, this gate may be tough. If either is true for you, please reach out and get help. We believe everything can be healed, including relationships with the Divine Masculine, so please find the courage to work with a professional. Allowing yourself to fully embody your Divine Feminine energy is a rite (and right) of passage in birth and most of us need that powerful, supportive and loving presence of a sacred birth partner to really step into that Mother Goddess self.

Let Go of Independence

Most modern-day women have a tendency to do it all on their own. It's what we expect from ourselves and what society expects from us too. The pressure is intense. And we all do a pretty great job of balancing this circus act called life as strong independent women. But labor and birth are different. They require co-dependency. Yes, of course, we can do it on our own, but do we really want to?

A big part of this gate is learning to let go of our independence and learn how to accept co-dependence when it is appropriate and healthy. The Gatekeeper knows the only way the Maiden Goddess is going to do just that is if she takes away her ability to walk. She has to sacrifice the one thing that keeps her on her own. When the Maiden Goddess realizes crawling won't cut it, she is forced to look for help outside of herself. Labor brings us to the same place. It can be scary, vulnerable, intimidating, shameful, and a whole other mix of emotions. But it is necessary to learn to cross this threshold. This is why having a dedicated and trustworthy Sacred Partner—one who can embody the Divine Masculine—is such a powerful way to cross this gate. When we trust and love our birth partners, it is so much easier to be carried without fighting it. There is less resistance, and we may even unexpectedly find comfort in the co-dependency, just like the Maiden Goddess.

Nothing is Forever

We've found that one of the best ways to lean toward co-dependency, especially if this is difficult on a personal level, is to realize that nothing lasts forever. The Maiden Goddess knows that she may need to be carried for a while, but as soon as she regains her strength and heals a bit, she will walk again on her own. This truth can help you to surrender to being carried across the threshold of this gate. It's time to let go of doing it all on your own and allow your Sacred Partner to hold the space and carry you through the labor emotionally, spiritually, energetically, and perhaps even very literally. The journal prompts below and the other Integration Practices can help you find a deeper connection to your own experience and help work out any hang-ups around this gate.

Honor the Fatherhood Journey

If the father is part of the birth process, it is very important to honor his journey as well so that he can fully step into his Divine Masculine energy, especially if he is your sacred birth partner too. Just like you are going through the transition from Maiden-to-Mother, dad is taking a similar journey. He is shedding his old-self and moving into his new Father-self. He has to walk through his own Gates of Transformation and with that comes a wide variety of emotions, realizations, fears, shames, expectations, and more. As moms, if we honor the fatherhood journey, we can actually create deeper intimacy and trust in the Divine Masculine while we labor.

But this means we have to hold space in pregnancy for the wounded parts of our partner so they can be expressed and healed. This is no easy task when we are overwhelmed with our own journey. On our website, www.laborlikeagoddess.com, we have some courses that can help couples navigate this tricky relationship as well as an e-book just for dads to help them fully step into their Divine Masculine energy.

INTEGRATION PRACTICES

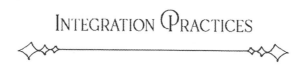

The following practices are intended to help you integrate the information of this chapter and apply it to your life now, so you can prepare to walk through this gate with trusted codependence when you're in labor. Take your time going through the practices that resonate the most with you and feel free to do them as often as you'd like.

SELF-LOVE ACTIVITY: YOUR OWN DIVINE SELF

One of the best ways to prepare for this gate is to recognize your own Divine Feminine and Divine Masculine as well as your own wounded feminine and wounded masculine self.

To do this, fold a piece of paper in half and in half again, so that you end up with four equal squares. In each square, add the following labels: "My Divine Feminine," "My Divine Masculine," "My Wounded Feminine," and "My Wounded Masculine."

Spend a few minutes focusing on each and writing down the qualities you have. Generally, the qualities we like about ourselves are divine, and the qualities we don't like about ourselves are wounded. Write down as many as you can think of. Then take a look at the paper. What do you notice? What do you feel when you see your personality divided in this way? Where do you have the most qualities? Spend some time journaling about this.

SELF-LOVE ACTIVITY: CALLING ON YOUR TRIBE

On a piece of paper, write down every family member and friend who would be willing to help in some way—even if only small—during pregnancy, labor, and postpartum. On another piece of paper, write down all the needs you anticipate having as you step into motherhood. Some ideas are meal trains, rides to doctor's appointments, babysitting, cleaning, emotional support, and so on. Start to preliminarily assign these "jobs" to those who are willing to help and then ask for their help. If you find this difficult, go ahead and explore the journal prompts below.

INNER EXPLORATION JOURNAL PROMPTS

The following journal prompts are for you to explore and uncover the different challenges of this gate. The practice of journaling can be deeply healing and enlightening, so we encourage you to spend some time reading over the prompts to see which ones resonate with you. Look back at these often. You might notice that different journal prompts resonate at different times.

Asking for Help

- Do I have a difficult time asking for help? Why or why not?
- How do I feel when others help me?
- What do I believe it says about my character if I ask for or receive help?
- Do I prefer to do everything on my own? If so, why?
- Do I easily receive help from others when offered? Why or why not?
- What would it mean if I actually asked more often for help? How would my life change? What feelings would I have to face?
- Who in my life would be willing to help me during pregnancy, labor, and postpartum and who have I yet to ask for help?
- What areas in life do I anticipate needing help? During labor? Needing food? Cleaning? Babysitting? Emotional support? Spiritual help? Who can I ask to help?
- If I could have an ideal helping situation, what would it look like?
- How can I practice receiving more easily before labor begins?

Understanding the Divine Masculine

- What does the Divine Masculine represent for me?

- What qualities do I think of when I think of God embodied in a person?
- What was my relationship like with my own father? Does that reflect how I feel about the masculine?
- Was my father more in his wounded masculine or Divine Masculine energy?
- Did my father make me feel safe and protected, or vulnerable and exposed?
- Do I trust the Divine Masculine?
- Can I tell the difference between the Divine Masculine and wounded masculine in myself and in others?
- Who will be the Divine Masculine energy at my birth? How will I ask them? Will I offer to let them participate in the co-creation of my Energetic Birth Plan? Why or why not?
- Do I trust my appointed Divine Masculine energy to advocate for me in a way that will make me feel empowered? If not, how can I adjust this? Who in my life right now can hold the space of the Divine Masculine for me in labor?

Sense of Safety

- What makes me feel safe when I am vulnerable?
- What qualities within the Divine Masculine make me feel safe?
- What can someone say to me to help me feel better when I'm scared? What words of reassurance seem to always work? What things can someone say to make it worse?
- What can I say to myself when I feel mistrusting, scared, or unsure of the path forward? What smells bring me a sense of safety? Do I want to use these during intense moments in labor?

Embracing Co-dependence

- What are my stories around co-dependency? How does embracing co-dependence make me feel?
- Has co-dependence been a healthy or unhealthy expression in my life and family?

- Do I have a good example in my life of healthy co-dependence?
- Do I have a good example in my life of unhealthy co-dependence?
- Do I fear the intimacy and vulnerability of letting myself become co-dependent? If so, why do I think that is?
- Can my sacred birth partner make me feel safe in co-dependence during labor in birth? Why or why not?

GODDESS RITUAL: OPENING YOUR THROAT CHAKRA

What You Need:

- A song you know by heart
- Some privacy
- Courage

What to Do:

This ritual might seem silly, but one of the hardest parts of asking for help can be getting the words out. This ritual will help you to open up your throat chakra (see Chapter 1) and get your vocal cords moving. This ritual can be done alone or with your partner. Get in a car, the shower, or in a smaller room in your home and pick your favorite song to belt out. Everyone has one. Something you know all the words to. Blast that music and SING! Rock out! Sing this song over and over again until you feel like you can feel your voice set free. Afterward, approach your partner and tell them what you need from them. See how the words just roll right off your tongue.

GODDESS RITUAL: MAIDEN-TO-MOTHER AFFIRMATION

Say the following affirmation as often as you like aloud, quietly or as a mantra over and over again as you transition from Maiden-to-Mother. Place your hands over your throat chakra and say: *"I open my mind, body, and soul to receive the help given by others. I am strong when I use my voice to ask for help!"*

THRESHOLD MEDITATION

In this meditation, you'll go on a short journey through the Gate of Sacred Partnership to enter into your more trusting self. This is a perfect meditation if you have been struggling to ask for help and surrender to the Divine Masculine. This practice can be done after each journal prompt or daily until you feel complete in your transition. It is also a great meditation for labor when those moments of mistrust and resistance show up. Visit www.laborlikeagoddess.com to download it.

Final Thoughts

This can be one of the hardest gates to walk through in labor because we're just not used to feeling safe enough to surrender to the masculine, even if it is Divine. But doing the work in this book, walking through each of the gates, and preparing ahead of time with a compassionate and conscious birth partner can set yourself up for a successful surrender and allow yourself to be carried through with the supportive and loving energy of the Divine Masculine. As you get more in touch with your own inner masculine and feminine sides, you will find it much easier to connect with those energies in others. Doing so will make it easier to allow yourself be carried through this gate!

CHAPTER VII

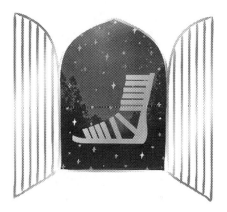

THE GATE OF FORTITUDE

MANAGING LABOR PAIN

Sometimes life will kick you around, but sooner or later you realize you aren't just a survivor. You are a warrior, and you are stronger than anything life throws your way.

—*Brooke Davis*

The Maiden Goddess and her beloved arrived at the next gate and much to her relief, she could walk again—it was just a temporary sacrifice of independence. So, she climbed down from her beloved's arms and realized that the locket was indeed NOT temporary and felt its immense weight against her heart. She was still fully embodied, she wasn't going to get off that easy, but she was also pretty used to it by now.

At first, the Maiden Goddess thought they had arrived at the wrong gate because this one wasn't like the rest. It was made of rickety, dilapidated wood and looked as if it would fall over if she leaned against it. But it too was enchanted, so she had to knock—hoping her beloved hadn't taken her off the path.

As soon as she knocked, another old Gatekeeper appeared and surveyed the two of them. She asked, "What business do you have knocking on my gate?"

The Maiden Goddess said with revived energy, "I long to become a mother. I wish to go to the Underworld."

"Ah, I see," said the Gatekeeper. "Then you will need to walk through this gate. And you will need to give me those shoes you are wearing. I could use a pair like that for what lies beyond this gate."

"What lies ahead?" the Maiden Goddess wondered. She looked down at her feet, the only part of her body that was still protected in some way. She then looked into her beloved's eyes, knowing that she could turn back with him and give up her quest, give up the heaviness of the locket, and go back to her sun-filled world. They could run away from it all. But her longing to become a mother just wouldn't let her, so she agreed to sacrifice her shoes.

As soon as she handed over her shoes, the Gatekeeper said, "Oh and you will have to say goodbye to your beloved. This next part is just for you."

She looked at her beloved, thanked him, and watched him walk away. The gates opened, and the Maiden Goddess immediately understood just how different this gate was. What appeared on the other side was not the familiar rocky path she was so used to seeing, but rather a long descent of spiraling stairs, each with broken shards of glass scattered on them.

Rage pulsed through her veins as she gazed upon this staircase of pain. "No . . . This isn't fair!" The Maiden screamed, "This is NOT what we agreed to. How am I supposed to get down those stairs without my shoes and being fully embodied! It will be excruciating! I did not sign up for this kind of suffering . . . You tricked me. . . If I would have known . . ." Her rants trailed off. The Maiden Goddess felt betrayed by the Gatekeeper. She longed for her beloved to come to rescue her.

The Gatekeeper, rather calmly, replied, "This is the sacrifice required. You will just have to learn to make friends with pain."

The Maiden Goddess knew there was no turning back now, and she could see how much pain awaited her on those stairs. The anticipation struck fear in her heart, yet she knew the only way through, was down. So, she took her first excruciating step.

It truly was a descent into the darkness and into her own inner darkness. Each step was more excruciating than the last. Each step more emotionally overwhelming. Glass lodged into her feet, spilling blood everywhere, making it slippery to find her footing. At one point, she fell and glass lodged along one side of her body. Tears streamed down her face, and she wanted to give up. Would this ever end? She couldn't see the end of the staircase—was there even one? When would this be over? Was this just a cruel joke? Could someone please save her!

She started to fear her own mind and saw herself succumbing to despair and suffering. She pulled a piece of glass out of her foot and caught her reflection in it. She gazed upon her defeated face. At that moment, she knew that the battle was not with the stairs, but was within herself. She knew that to overcome the pain, she had to become it, for the pain was her, and she was the pain. There was no separation except the one her mind wanted to make.

She boldly proclaimed, "Hear me now mind, body, spirit. I am stronger than I believe at this moment and the power of the thousands of mothers that came before me pumps through my veins. I descend these stairs with every other mother, and with their strength. I will not just survive, I will thrive. I choose to lean in. I choose to become this experience. Not separate from it."

The moment she declared this and knew it in her heart, she melted into the experience and no longer felt any pain. Instead, she noticed a euphoria come over her and a deep sense of inner strength and connection to herself and her baby. This connection empowered her to press on, and before she knew it, she made it to the bottom of those goddess-forsaken stairs!

A Different Kind of Gate

This gate is the main gate of labor, or at least the one that most pregnant moms are concerned with and prepare for ahead of time. So, we may recognize much about this gate if we've already been doing the work to prepare by reading books, taking childbirth classes, learning comfort measures and laboring positions, practicing breathing techniques, doing hypnosis, hiring doulas, saying affirmations, getting epidurals, administering medications, and so forth. We do all this because we know this is the gate where we will have to face pain and lean into many, very intense 60–90-second contractions over and over and over again, for hours, sometimes days on end, all to birth our babies. Developing fortitude is what is asked of us as we transition into motherhood.

What we may not realize is that through all this preparation, we are only preparing for the *first* sacrifice that this gate asks of us: the sacrifice of our metaphorical shoes so we can face our physical pain. But this gate doesn't stop at one sacrifice. To make it through, we are asked to sacrifice over and over and over again by facing our emotional, spiritual, and psychological pain at the same time as the physical pain. And it is these multiple and simultaneous sacrifices that can catch us off guard if we don't fully understand what this gate requires of us. So much of current childbirth preparation does laboring women a disservice by not speaking about the multiple types of pain that show up in labor. Hopefully, by the end of this chapter, you will feel prepared and be able to recognize them as they show up for you.

The Maiden Shows Us the Way Through

The Maiden Goddess in our story is just like most laboring moms. We tend to assume we know how things are going to go at the beginning of the journey, and no matter how many times we've given birth, we are usually surprised that things don't go the way we thought. Every birth is different, and all births have elements of surprise, especially if we have strong expectations. (see Chapter 4). When the Maiden Goddess approaches the Gate of Fortitude, she assumes that the sacrifice of the shoes will be enough to get her through the gate, as perhaps it may have been before. But in reality, the shoes are just the first sacrifice that opens the door to much more sacrifice. Labor is the same way. We are often prepared to open ourselves up to a certain level of sensation and think that it will stay at that level the entire labor. We think, "Okay, I'm showing up. I'm making the sacrifice," and then look for the end. But in labor, the first sacrifice is never the end and, just like the Maiden Goddess, when we see that gate swing open, and that endless spiral staircase full of glass appears, we can often panic, move into a fear–pain cycle, disembody (as described in Chapter 5), or resort to a whole slew of other coping mechanisms that get us stuck.

This is why, as doulas, we've heard more often than not, women proclaim in utter surprise when their labor picks up, "I knew it was going to be painful, but I didn't know it was going to be *this* painful! I didn't think it would be *this* hard!" We believe the "this" in each statement refers to that metaphorical and painful staircase in the story. We've also come to observe that it's not so much the physical sensation these women are referring to but rather the experience of being faced with all the types of pain at once—emotional, spiritual, and psychological pain PLUS the physical sensation on repeat for hours. Feeling all pain on all levels of being is an all-encompassing and overwhelming experience that seldom presents itself outside of labor. It is a foreign and bizarre experience. We usually aren't mentally or emotionally prepared for this level of intensity, and we can't recognize what it is as it happens. But this chapter is designed to help you understand this gate and get to the level of preparation where you feel you can descend your own stairs in labor.

Labor is unique and very different from everyday life. We are not usually asked to make repeated sacrifices without a known end in sight. On the contrary, there is usually a final destination that we can linearly and logically map out. We usually can see the whole journey and what it's going to take to reach the end goal from the very beginning. For example, with the journey to getting a college degree, we know ahead of time the sacrifices that may be required—four years of schooling, late nights studying, a set financial debt amount, saying no to fun, and exercising the mind—all of these are self-contained sacrifices that can be anticipated. But the Gate of Fortitude teaches how to sacrifice when the end isn't in sight, and when we don't know the intensity, duration, or number of sacrifices.

This can feel scary, overwhelming, and too much. The moment when we are faced with this intensity is often the moment that mamas who wanted to go "all-natural" call out for pain relief from the overwhelm— it's just too much to handle. Or in another scenario, we had a laboring mama in transition—the moment right before the pushing stage—declare to the medical staff and us that today was not going to be the day she was going to have a baby. She then very determinedly got up off the bed and started to walk home. Within taking a few steps down the hallway, she surrendered and was pushing, but this story goes to show how old coping mechanisms can take over when we are overwhelmed. Hers was complete denial!

And this isn't a bad thing. Even the Maiden Goddess calls out to be saved from the experience—it's a truly natural instinct to run, hide, ignore, deny, disembody, etc., when we feel overwhelmed. It is how we cope in real life, but labor is different, and just like the Maiden Goddess who chooses not to run away, you will also find yourself faced with the opportunity to walk through this gate. Instead of resisting the experience, you can choose to begin your descent down the stairs, choose more sacrifice, more vulnerability, more courage, and more strength—even to the point where you may not—and probably won't—have anything left to give. Fortitude can only be developed from this place, and the Maiden Goddess shows us how to cultivate the strength of character to *lean in*to the sensations, rather than feel victimized so we can walk through this gate with dignity and empowerment. She teaches us that *how* we experience this gate is completely our choice.

The Symbolism of the Gate

Let's learn more about the Maiden Goddess' process through the symbolism of the various elements in the story.

The Dilapidated Wooden Gate

The gate looks different than the previous ones. It is rickety and appears as if it will fall over. This is a very important visual symbol because pain—whether physical, emotional, or psychological—often looks less foreboding than it actually is, and we can easily underestimate its power over us. We can think it's an old gate that can topple over with our will power but then we are sorely mistaken once we are in its throes. Pain in labor is tricky and powerful like that.

The gate isn't a strong, heavy, iron door that can be propped open and walked right through just once. Rather, this gate swings both ways and may even hit us as we're walking through it. In labor, pain can feel this way too, as if some invisible wind blows it back and forth through our bodies, each time hitting a new threshold of intensity. This can be alarming if we are expecting only one or two blows.

As humans, we often underestimate pain when we aren't in it, and then once we are in it, to cope with it, we can let ourselves become victimized by it—begging for relief or to be saved from it. But the reason this gate swings back and forth, over and over, is because pain is trying to teach us not to resist it, but to lean into it. And that is because the pain in labor is not truly pain—it is a sensation that we have taught ourselves to call pain because we have no other frame of reference. But our goal is that by the end of this chapter, we will all be able to show that "pain in labor" is really what happens when we have physical intensity plus emotional resistance to the experience. We, like the Maiden, become the experience rather than resist it and so walk through this Gate of Fortitude with a newly defined strength of character and the high probability of experiencing the antithesis of pain—the pleasure of birth.

The Shoes

Just as real shoes protect our feet from the ground, the metaphorical shoes in the story represent the things we hold on to emotionally, physically, and psychologically to keep our egos and bodies protected from pain. Pain has become a four-letter profanity in our society, and we seem to do everything we can to avoid, numb, medicate, resist, and block it. But pain is an essential part of the human experience, and whenever we try to escape a part of our experience, we inevitably create more pain for ourselves in the long run.

In our story, the shoes protect the Maiden's feet from the rocky path so she can walk all the way to the Underworld pain-free and as efficiently as possible. It's reasonable to believe that without her shoes, she will get injured, which might prevent her mission from being successful. It is a big ask to sacrifice her shoes. The Maiden knows that by handing over her shoes, she is making herself vulnerable to injury and pain.

So, when she is asked to hand over essential tools she needs, it just doesn't add up in the Maiden's mind. She is giving up the last remnants of the protection she brought with her and thus deepening her courage and vulnerability. She also has to face the fear that she could very well not make it and accept that her expectations of how or if she will arrive in motherhood may not be met. She is also being asked to deepen her trust in the journey, the calling in her heart and the choices she is making, thereby strengthening her sovereignty. So, by the time she hands over her shoes, it's as if she has walked through the first three gates all at once all over again! No wonder this gate feels painful!

This is such a beautiful metaphor for what is asked of us with each contraction of labor. It's as if we are asked to be vulnerable, courageous, trusting, and sovereign all at once with each wave of the uterus. We are asked to move through multiple gates with every 60–90-second surge, every few minutes. It takes the ability to labor like a goddess to embrace this energy rather than fight against it, which is why it is so important to practice walking through these gates before labor really begins and our skills are put to the test, under intense pressure.

The Maiden may not have been capable or mature enough to walk through this gate and give up her shoes if she didn't have the experience of the previous gates and didn't recognize the rewards that come after the sacrifices... she may have given up. But she knew that by sacrificing her sword (protection against fear), she had gained courage and true sovereignty over her emotions. By sacrificing her cloak (the ability to play small and hide), she had gained expansion through vulnerability, and by sacrificing her map (her expectations), she had learned trust. Just like the Maiden Goddess, we too need to walk through the gates as much as we can ahead of time, experience the rewards that come with our willing sacrifice, and condition ourselves to the habit of effortless and graceful transformation.

The Spiral Stairs of Pain

Let's talk about the symbolism of the staircase, because no other gate has this peculiar feature. The Maiden doesn't get to waltz through the gate once she's made her sacrifice. Instead, what appears is more sacrifice in the form of a spiraling staircase with glass shards on each step, descending into the abyss of darkness, with no end in sight. Sounds like a horror movie! And in a way, it kind of is because it stirs up all kinds of fear and anticipation within us.

From the top of the steps, we can imagine the emotions that hit the Maiden Goddess as she stares at the journey ahead. She's just given up her shoes and thought she was walking through the gate only to discover a new journey—one that looks incredibly painful. It's this fear of anticipation that can get us in trouble before we even begin our descent because it can trap us in the infamous fear-pain cycle.

We talked a lot about the fear–pain cycle in Chapter 1 and how it can increase the intensity of pain which then, in turn, increases our fear, and round and round we go, trapped in an endless cycle that can ultimately lead to suffering. The moment we enter suffering, we've lost our ability to choose to be vulnerable, courageous, sovereign, and strong—endangering all our progress so far. Anticipation, if we let it, can be the starter match for this fear–pain cycle.

Even the Maiden Goddess, for a moment, falls prey to this tempting offer. Before she even starts her descent, she blames the Gatekeeper for lying to her, complains that it isn't fair, and starts to fall victim to the experience, rather than being empowered by it. We've seen many laboring women start to point blame as soon as labor intensifies. But as we learned in previous chapters, when we point blame, we lose our sovereignty, fall victim to the experience, and easily disembody. The Maiden Goddess remembers this and recognizes that with each sacrifice comes reward, and that is enough encouragement to help her reject the temptation to cope, and instead, begin her descent into greater sacrifice.

The first of many sacrifices asked on this staircase becomes apparent after she descends a few steps. Just like in labor, the Maiden Goddess experiences a compounding effect of the sensation and emotion with each stair. Without an end in sight, she must walk blindly with a pain that intensifies with each step, which asks for a deeper and deeper surrender simultaneously. This is a beautiful metaphor for how the nature of labor progresses.

It is also very different from how we experience *pain* in other situations. Usually, we get one solid blow that shoots pain messages to our brain, and over time, the pain lessens as our body heals. There is an intensity followed by a relief. Think about stubbing your toe. At first, there is intense pain, but we know if we "wait it out," it will go away. But throughout labor, time means more intensity, not less. Yes, there are breaks in between contractions when moms can even fall asleep, but expect the overall movement of labor to be one of intensification, not relief until the baby is born. Once the baby is out, all the sensation of pain transmutes into love instantly. If we have learned to cope with pain in our everyday life by waiting for it to subside after some time, labor can feel traumatic and overwhelming when this doesn't happen. However, if we prepare ourselves for this compounding effect, we can recognize it when it shows up in our labor and, just like the Maiden Goddess, lean into those shards of glass.

Because in all reality, the "pain" we are experiencing is our own body. It's a way of looking at our reflection in the glass shards. We can choose to stop being the victim of our body's sensations and our emotions, and instead lean in and melt with it. Just like the Maiden Goddess, when we do this, we significantly reduce the sensation of pain and can even transmute it into euphoria. It is this "becoming" that is how she masters the descent.

In all the labors we have witnessed, no matter the circumstance, the women who choose to lean into their sensations—open deeper into the experience and invite their emotions to be witnessed and acknowledged— are the ones who have the most empowered, successful transformations. Sometimes just the simple act of relaxing the jaw can make this "becoming" possible and provide the opportunity to labor like a goddess and descend the stairs of pain with strength and serenity. The women who resist the sensations and feelings tend to walk away from their labor experiences feeling unsatisfied, disappointed, and sometimes even traumatized by it.

This gate is asking us to go deeper when we labor. This is why the staircase is a spiral rather than linear because it keeps coming back around to the same place, just at a deeper level each time. This is truly the spiraling energy of labor. Contractions get stronger and more intense as time goes on, not lighter and easier. Each surge of pressure is a deepening of intensity rather than a lightening up. Because the sensations and emotions in labor only deepen, if we resist one level of the staircase, when that comes back around even deeper, we can feel extremely overwhelmed and overpowered by our own bodies.

This is because laboring women often try to just "get through" a contraction rather than "getting washed away with it." The difference is that in one scenario, the mother is looking to relieve her pain, while in the other, she surrenders to the intensity and becomes the pain. This is a very important distinction that can only be understood once we learn how to walk through the gates. When we trust the benefits that come with the sacrifice, we can more willingly lean in. This is one of the reasons we feel so strongly that learning to walk through the gates ahead of time is one of the best pain-management techniques any woman can learn.

But as we will see in the next section, pain in labor isn't real pain, so the same rules don't apply. When we go into labor thinking it's going to ease up, we can set ourselves up to be overwhelmed and disappointed. Birth is a descent into compounded sensation. So, we step on the first shard of glass, and if we cope using "time," we often find ourselves suffering because, just like the Maiden Goddess, we can't see the bottom. The only way to get to the end is to take one step at a time, without relying on the comfort of "how much longer." This can be a terrifying prospect for women who don't prepare for this ahead of time and it can often lead to victimization and suffering in labor. So, the best way to cope with the stairs of pain is to lean in. And the best way to lean in is to really understand that sensation in labor is only pain if we choose to define it as such.

What Is Pain Really?

Pain is an unpleasant feeling or sensation interpreted by the brain through sensory neurons signaling actual or potential injury to the body. These signals are not just physical but rely on subjective information and perception for the brain to interpret. On top of all of that, various unconscious and conscious responses to the sensation and the perception of it, including emotional response, add to the meaning of the pain by the brain. So, in short, pain is made up of physical, emotional, and psychological meanings.

Pain also isn't linear. It ebbs and flows. It surges and retreats. It throbs and stabs or radiates or dulls. Pain changes and shifts, and that is what makes it sometimes easier to deal with because we know it won't last forever unless we tell ourselves something else. The perception of our pain and the meaning we give to that perception are just as much responsible for our level of pain as the physical sensation itself—in labor, even more so.

This is because labor pain isn't pain. According to this definition, pain is derived from a signal of actual or potential injury to the body— for example, when we get a cut or a burn or pull a muscle. Our body signals to the brain that we are injured and we can react appropriately. But labor contractions are not injurious to the body—it is the natural flexing of the uterus muscle, so labor is more like the burn of working out than the pain of breaking an arm. But we use the word "pain" to describe the sensation, even though nothing wrong is happening in the body. Why?

We believe that it wasn't always this way. As we mentioned in previous chapters, in the societies where birth was a natural part of everyday life, women experienced much less fear, shame, and expectations about birth and therefore their experiences were more pleasurable and fulfilling. But as we started to define birth as scary and dangerous and took away a woman's sovereignty in knowing her own body and her own sensations, "pain" became a normal word in labor. But it doesn't have to be that way and many brave women who trust their bodies and their babies are proving the status quo wrong by having pain-free births every day. It's just not as exciting to watch a woman on TV having a peaceful birth, so we don't hear about it very often. But as doulas, we can tell you that more often than not, women are learning to walk through these Gates of Transformation despite all the obstacles meant to keep them disempowered and are changing the game in birth! And we all can have this amazing experience.

It starts with redefining what we call "pain" in birth with other more accurate words like "sensation," "pressure," "intensity," "burn," "opening," "softening," and "melting." We can even take the suggestion of hypnobirthing and use the word "surge" to define a contraction to give a more accurate visualization of what is happening in the labor process. It's also important to be honest with ourselves about the emotional pain we are experiencing and use more accurate words to describe what is happening for us on an emotional level like "overwhelm," "fear," "disappointment," "panic," and "vulnerability." When we don't use accurate words for describing the sensations and just use the blanket term, we are actually telling our body that something is really wrong, triggering all the defense mechanisms and emotions that go along with this level of alarm—fear, fight-flight-freeze, resistance, restriction, etc., —increasing our adrenaline and anxiety.

But, if we change how we talk about birth and truly understand what is happening on a physical, emotional, and spiritual level, we can lean into the sensations, deepen our vulnerability to the process and cultivate inner strength. We can allow ourselves to develop these natural calluses so that, just like the Maiden Goddess, we never needed our metaphorical shoes to begin with.

Who Is Birthing Whom?

One of the best ways to lean in as a laboring mother is to truly understand that we don't birth our babies. They birth themselves. We are merely the vessel that provides a safe, happy, peaceful, and open opportunity for our babies to make their big debut into the world. Whenever we tell moms this in labor, it shifts the energy dramatically. All of a sudden, understanding that our only job as laboring women is to open ourselves up for our babies and get out of their way becomes much more of a reasonable task. Things like pain and sacrifice become secondary to the calling of giving our babies an obstacle-free experience. It's as if the responsibility and pressure to "birth our babies" can get in the way of our labors when all we really have to do is surrender to the babies.

That's because our babies are in charge. They control how fast and intense or slow and steady the labor is. They are the ones who signal to the uterus to contract and at what pace, intensity, and duration. The babies are the ones who know what is going on inside of the womb, so it only makes sense that they are the ones at the wheel. Perhaps the cord is wrapped around too tightly, and so the baby needs three strong and long contractions, even though there have already been many like it before, so they can move the cord out of the way. Or perhaps the baby isn't in the right position to come down the birth canal, so they signal to the uterus to surge soft then hard then soft then hard, so they can maneuver into the perfect position for over four hours. As much as we'd like to take the credit, we are really just along for the ride as our babies control the entire labor.

As they should! It is their first big effort, and it's also the first co-created activity with mom. We've already had our own births where we were at the wheel. Now it's the baby's turn. So as mothers, we can choose to resist our labors, thereby making it more difficult for our babies to do what they need to do, OR we can surrender and trust that our babies have good reasons for why they need to move quicker or slower and support our babies in their creative efforts to be born.

Most women truly want to support their babies and make their children feel loved, empowered, and nurtured in every activity they attempt. It's part of mothering to uplift our kid's efforts. The only thing that usually gets in the way of doing just that is the unconscious resistance to our own Gates of Transformation. This is why we felt it was so important to write this book to help women understand that our only job in labor is to walk through our own gates, so our babies have the easiest, most open path to being born.

However, the Gate of Fortitude can be one of the hardest to surrender to, and it can make it really easy to ask for that epidural when we don't want it, or escape old coping mechanisms. But if we can remember that each step on those metaphorical glass-covered stairs is a deepening that actually makes it that much easier for our babies to have a clear way, we can find the courage and strength to lean into it . . . for them. Hopefully understanding this spiritual and physical process that happens in labor can give us even more permission to walk through this gate with empowerment.

Having an Empowered Epidural

We've mentioned how epidurals can be unconsciously used as an escape mechanism or as a way to avoid a Gate of Transformation. But for others, having an epidural can be the most empowered and embodied way to labor. There are so many circumstances where this is true and is done with so much consciousness, awareness, and sovereignty that we wanted to take a moment and honor this amazing choice in labor. We believe that any choice as long as it is made with consciousness and sovereignty is the best choice for mama and baby.

For moms-to-be with unresolved sexual trauma or boundary violations, an epidural is a very empowering way to have a vaginal birth rooted in love and openness. Epidurals are also powerful tools for mamas who don't have a strong support system or a Sacred Partner (see Chapter 6) to hold the space of the Divine Masculine, and must therefore do it themselves. And of course, if specific medical conditions arise before or during labor, epidurals can be the perfect choice for a safe and relaxed birth experience.

The keys to creating an empowered epidural birth are through understanding, awareness, and being embodied. In Appendix IV, we've included *Doula Tips to Have an Empowered Epidural Birth* to help a laboring mom do just that. These tips will help avoid some of the pitfalls that can happen with epidurals to knock us out of consciousness and into victimization.

With an epidural, we often remove the physical sensation of the uterus contracting, which can make it tempting to skip this gate. But, as we've already learned over and over again, when we skip or avoid or deny ourselves a gate, we can find ourselves dissatisfied with our birth experience. This is why it is most important for moms who are bedridden and physically numb to focus on their gates with greater intention and motivation. We've witnessed how skipping the Gate of Fortitude due to an epidural can delay the Maiden-to-Mother transition and set up greater challenges in postpartum. We've also seen it play out in a physical way where mom becomes so disembodied that contractions slow down or stop completely and more medical interventions are required to keep up labor and keep the baby safe.

So, to avoid these pitfalls, walk through the Gate of Fortitude, and face the other types of pain that are asking to be felt. Focus on staying in your body through breath, movement, and intention. Connect with the baby even more deeply and let him/her/them know that you are present and in your body, that you have not abandoned yourself or baby and that you are holding loving space. Redirect your energy to fulfilling your Energetic Birth Plan (see Chapter 4). Bring love and laughter into the space. Find gratitude and reverence for the birth. Cherish your last moments of maidenhood.

As mentioned in a previous chapter, pre- and perinatal psychology are proving that *how* we are born into the world sets the stage for our entire personality. When a baby is born from an empowered and conscious epidural, they are born into love. However, if an epidural brings disempowerment to mom, the baby is also affected and may end up having emotional and psychological wounding around feeling victimized or abandoned. This is why we feel that those with epidurals have an even greater calling to lean into all the gates with intention, embodiment, love, and determination.

Pain as Energy

When we have any kind of pain that shows up in labor, it is helpful to understand what pain is from an energetic and spiritual standpoint. Pain is nothing more than stuck energy, or chi, in the body, aura, or chakra system. When energy gets stuck, it starts to bottleneck in certain areas, and as that energy builds, our brain perceives it as greater pain. And energy can get stuck anywhere—in our minds, auras, chakras, or physical body.

This is also how emotional pain develops. The emotion gets stuck, becomes very intense and will often bleed over into the physical body causing physical pain as well. We've learned that fear lives in the first chakra, so when fear builds up and gets stuck and can no longer flow properly, it becomes emotionally painful and can manifest in the organs around the first chakra—bladder, anus, or vagina, for example. Often times constipation is a direct result of a build-up of fear in the first chakra— a fear of releasing and letting go that manifests as a physical holding on to waste. The same is true for shame in the second chakra, which affects the womb and hips; and for the power struggle of expectations in the third chakra affecting the stomach, liver, and pancreas Understanding our emotions and where they sit in our body can give us insight to the discomfort we are feeling in labor and in life.

When pain shows up in labor, it's good to investigate where the energy is stuck, the affected chakra, and then use a few simple techniques to help return flow to the area. This is one of the reasons that acupuncture in pregnancy and labor is such a useful tool. The needles bring the energy flow back to stuck areas, thereby helping with pain management.

Energetic tools do wonders too! At the end of this chapter, there is a simple visualization technique that can be used on areas of pain, or anywhere there is a sensation of stuck energy. This can be incredibly helpful, especially when we find ourselves resisting a gate, fighting a surge, or trying to escape the pain experience. Many mothers who have used these tools found their pain to be very minimal throughout labor. We also highly recommend teaching your Sacred Partner these tools to help guide you in those moments of doubt and resistance throughout labor.

How to Walk Through the Gate of Fortitude

So, we have already mentioned that there are at least four different kinds of pain that you might experience in labor: physical, emotional, psychological, and spiritual pain. Understanding the differences between each of these can help you find appropriate and useful coping tools to deal with each aspect. But you need to be able to recognize what kind of pain you are experiencing first.

Let's start with physical pain. We already know that physical pain signals to the brain that something is harmful, wrong, or in danger of potential injury. If our pain doesn't meet this criterion, we know it isn't physical pain. But if it does, then we can address it with medication, natural coping tools, massage, acupuncture, or energy work. With physical pain, there is usually a block in the energy flow of the body. The best way to heal physical pain is to restore the blood flow and circulation to the area or remove the block. In labor, when experiencing physical pain, movement and breath are beautiful ways to restore the flow to the blocked area, whether we are experiencing back labor or cramping or other blocks of energy flow. It is important to know that the moment the baby is born, those physical pains disappear because the baby is no longer applying pressure or blocking blood flow. This is where childbirth preparation classes, comfort measures, and laboring positions really shine, and they are 100 percent worth the time and commitment to learning. Check out the Recommend Resources in the back of the book for our favorite childbirth methods.

But many times, these coping mechanisms only help with physical pain. When we start to experience emotional pain, we need different coping mechanisms to get us through, and usually different ones than the ones we use daily. Emotional pain is the pain we experience at the heart level when we resist our own experience, judge ourselves, shame ourselves, or inflict emotional harm upon ourselves. Many times, emotional pain can manifest as physical pain, but only if we ignore it. If we are in tune with our own emotional wellbeing, we should be able to easily catch emotional pain as it shows up, which is why we endorse practicing this level of consciousness in pregnancy. In labor, emotional pain often comes in the form of anger, frustration, shame, fear, disappointment, and despair. If we start to feel these feelings, we know that we have entered into emotional pain.

The only way to handle emotional pain is to recognize that emotions are just emotions. They ebb and flow and shift and change, even when they are intense, they don't have the power to control us unless we allow them to. This is a big part of learning emotional maturity, which is a necessity when it comes to motherhood. We must be able to witness our emotions, feel them but not be ruled by them. It's tricky and takes practice to learn, which is why we highly recommend walking through the first few gates as often as you can before labor begins. It helps train our minds into emotional maturity, and sometimes we need professional support to teach ourselves how to do this. We highly recommend psychotherapy as a powerful way to get in touch with emotion, feel validation, and learn healthy coping techniques.

When emotions begin to spiral out of control, it is usually due to some level of psychological pain—the pain we experience when a rigid worldview and/or belief system is challenged by the reality we are experiencing in the present moment. We see it manifest in labor as blame, victimization, or the belief that we are not in control of our own reactions, thoughts, beliefs, and actions. Psychological pain is often seen at the Gate of Expectations, where we are asked to be flexible with our expectations of birth. This is because psychological pain is caused by rigidity, and labor is the experience of mutability. So, wherever we are rigid in our thinking, our assumptions, our expectations, and even our feelings, we will experience psychological pain.

A good way to notice this is to catch yourself if you start making black-and-white statements or thinking thoughts like, "I have to birth this way only" or "There is no way I'm going to labor like this for much longer." Another great way to see the seeds of psychological pain is to notice where you give up your sovereignty to someone else or where you start to blame the experience. This is a telltale sign that you're experiencing psychological pain.

Psychological pain can cause trauma in birth, but there is a really powerful way to deal with it, and that is to practice being flexible—in your mind, in your beliefs and in your understanding of the world. Trust is a big player in your ability to do this. Practicing trust and being flexible about how you think things should be are the salves to heal psychological pain.

Finally, spiritual pain is the most elusive, and certainly, the least talked about in labor but also in life. We don't comment much on the spiritual pain of transformation and of the death/rebirth cycle. But when we resist the natural flow of transformation, we can start to experience spiritual pain. Because spiritual pain exists on a soul level, it can take some time to filter down into our experience. But if we are sensitive to our own transformation, we can catch spiritual pain before it ever manifests. This is why it is so incredibly important to be aware of our own spiritual pain, so we don't inadvertently manifest something very difficult to heal. But to be aware of spiritual pain, we must be aware of ourselves as spiritual beings. If we lean more toward an atheistic world view and don't view ourselves as spiritual beings having a human experience, recognizing and seeing this type of pain will be difficult. But if we believe in our eternal spiritual nature—the one that lives beyond time, space, and physicality—we have greater ease in acknowledging and surrendering to our spirit's will.

In labor, when we don't recognize and address spiritual pain, or we fight the death/rebirth cycle, it can manifest as a failure to progress. There is no physical, emotional, or even psychological reason the labor has stopped, but it has. Often as doulas, we've seen this happen when women resist the death of the Maiden-self and in doing so cause so much spiritual pain that it stops the process of birth until the mother surrenders or, more likely the case, medicine intervenes.

For these reasons and many more, it is vital to understand what kind of pain we are experiencing in labor as well as where it comes from so we can deal with it through empowerment and sovereignty. Having this kind of awareness takes time and practice to really get to know ourselves. This is why we have such extensive journal prompts throughout this book so that we can each learn more about ourselves, so labor can become a welcomed experience of transformation.

Integration Practices

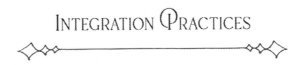

The following practices are intended to help you integrate the information of this chapter and apply it to your life now, so you can walk through this gate with fortitude while in labor! Take your time going through the practices that resonate the most with you and feel free to do them as often as you'd like.

SELF-LOVE ACTIVITY: VISUALIZATION TO RESTORE FLOW TO BLOCKED AREAS OF PAIN

This is an exercise you can start to use in pregnancy as your body stretches and opens with your growing uterus. Lie down in a comfortable place and give yourself at least 10 minutes of uninterrupted time by turning off your phone, closing the door and removing any other distractions. Take three deep breaths visualizing your spirit as a golden liquid light coming into your body through the top of your head and filling every space and every cell with liquid golden light. Notice where discomfort or pain arise. Without judgment, turn your attention to those areas and bathe them in that light. See if you can imagine any blocks or colors or symbols that relate to the pain. Imagine the golden light dissolving the blocks and restoring flow to the area. Don't worry if you don't get it all in one sitting. You can commit to doing this visualization often to bring more peace, love, and flow to your body and to practice greater embodiment. Share this visualization with your Sacred Partner so they too can guide you while in labor.

SELF-LOVE ACTIVITY: REFRAMING VOCABULARY

The purpose of this activity is to reframe any negative and pain-oriented words with positive and expansive words to describe the sensation. How you talk about your pain in labor can have a direct effect on how you experience it. Our words are very powerful. So, it is very important throughout the process to reframe the physical sensations, not as pain, but as a deep opening.

On a piece of paper, write down the phrases you use the most when you experience pain. Then, next to each phrase, write a more positive reframing, that you can start to practice. For example:

- Instead of "It hurts," how about "I am opening."
- Instead of "This is painful," how about "I am exploding into motherhood."
- Instead of "Ouch," how about "Ooohhhhhhh, yes."
- Instead of "No," how about "Yes."
- Instead of "I can't handle this," how about "I'm being stretched in love."

- Instead of "I can't do this," how about "I am stronger than I can even imagine."

Keep this list somewhere you can look at every day and spend time retraining your brain to see the positive. Your birth partner can help you remember to use more open, conscious words in labor as well.

SELF-LOVE ACTIVITY: GET TO KNOW YOUR INNER CHILD AND INVITE HER TO YOUR BIRTH

We all have an inner child that sometimes runs the show. She's the one who sometimes acts like a baby, throws tantrums, doesn't want to share, and thinks life is unfair. Whether you like it or not, your inner child is likely to show up at your birth experience because she always does when we experience transition. Because birth is so vulnerable and open AND it is a space of uber spiritual healing, our inner child wants to be healed and transmuted through this opportunity as well. So, if they are going to show up anyway and crash the party, we might as well offer an open-hearted invitation. Doing so can be very beneficial.

Some mamas actually write a letter or invitation to their inner child. Others like to visualize a conversation between themselves and their inner child. Whatever method works best for you, let your inner child know she can show up to your birth and sit quietly on a special chair. Some mamas will bring their old teddy bears or things that remind them of comfort in childhood to place on that chair in their laboring room. It's good to set up some ground rules with your inner child and let her know that she can speak up but can't throw a tantrum.

INNER EXPLORATION JOURNAL PROMPTS

The following journal prompts are for you to explore and uncover the different challenges of this gate. The practice of journaling can be deeply healing and enlightening, so we encourage you to spend some time reading over the prompts to see which ones resonate with you. Look back at these often. You might notice that different journal prompts resonate at different times.

Pain

- Do I understand the difference between my physical pain, psychological pain, spiritual pain, and emotional pain? If so, how do I know? If not, why not?
- How do I currently deal with each aspect of pain?
- What are things that I do to numb myself from pain or avoid pain?
- Do I plan on doing this during labor? If not, why not?
- How do I plan on managing my physical pain in labor? Emotional pain? Spiritual pain? Psychological pain?
- What about pain in childbirth do I fear the most?
- Have I ever been trapped in a fear-pain cycle? If so, what happened? How did I get out of it? What did I learn about myself from experiencing that?
- Can I reframe the word pain into a sensation? Yes or no? Why or Why not?
- When I am experiencing pain, what emotions come up for me? How do I process those emotions?

Connecting With Baby

- Do I feel connected to my baby? Why or why not?
- What can I do to connect more with my baby?
- Do I want to allow my baby to be in control of my labor? How does that make me feel? What are ways I can support my baby throughout my labor?
- How does it make me feel to know that I need to just get out of my own way and my baby's way in labor?
- How does it make me feel that my only job in labor is to walk through the Gates of Transformation?
- Do I trust that my baby knows what is best for them in labor? Why or why not?
- Can I trust my baby's timing? Why or why not?

- How can I cultivate more strength of character so I can walk through this gate?
- What is my own personal definition of fortitude?
- How do I plan to remind myself of fortitude when I'm in labor?
- What kind of support do I need in this gate from myself and others?
- What reminders will be nice to have while I'm at this gate?
- How will I recognize this gate in my labor?

GODDESS RITUAL: LABOR PEP TALK

What You Need:

- Phone or recording device
- Some time alone

What to Do:

Grab your phone and hit record. Spend the next few minutes giving yourself a pep talk. It sounds a little silly, but the best way to move through pain is motivation: the motivation to prevail. It can be a few lines of, "I can do it, I got this" or a bunch of curses! Whatever gets you pumped and urges you on. You can have your birth partner join in on the fun, adding music or sound effects. Labor can be long, so create something entertaining to get you through it. Then listen to it often and play it while you are in labor. If anything, it'll give you a laugh when things get intense.

GODDESS RITUAL: MAIDEN-TO-MOTHER AFFIRMATION

Say the following affirmation as often as you like out loud, quietly, or as a mantra over and over again as you transition from Maiden-to-Mother. Place your hands over your third-eye chakra and say: _"I have the mental strength and fortitude to reframe my pain into pleasure at any moment in time!"_

THRESHOLD MEDITATION

In this meditation, you'll go on a short journey through this gate and down the stairs to alchemize pain into pleasure. This is the perfect meditation if you fear the pain of labor, or you know that you don't do particularly well when certain types of pain show up. This practice can be done after each journal prompt or daily until you feel complete in your transition. It is also a great meditation for pregnancy and labor when those moments of pain really hit in the moment. Visit www.laborlikeagoddess.com to download it.

Final Thoughts

We hope this chapter has helped you see pain in a completely different way and inspired you to approach your labor with a new set of eyes: ones that are flexible, compassionate, empowered, and aware. And through these eyes and through the practices we provide, you can find your own inner fortitude to face everything this gate asks you to sacrifice and know you can do it over and over and over until your baby is in your arms.

~ CHAPTER VIII ~

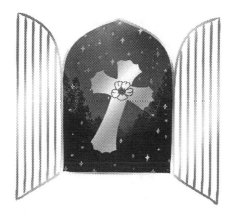

THE GATE OF INTENTIONAL SURRENDER
ACCEPTING SPIRITUAL DEATH

Life and death are not opposites; ego and life are opposites. Ego is against both life and death. The ego is afraid to live, and the ego is afraid to die. It is afraid to live because each effort, each step towards life, brings death closer.

—*Osho*

The Maiden Goddess collapsed in exhaustion and euphoria, as she reached the bottom of the stairs. She was overcome with a deep sense of pride in her perseverance, endurance, and fortitude. The last gate was truly mind over matter, and she felt such sovereignty over her own thoughts. As she focused on her rewards, her wounds started to heal miraculously, and she found herself standing up and walking forward. She could feel that her baby was almost within reach. She was very close to the center of the Underworld.

With this realization, a large crucifix magically appeared before her, with the last Gatekeeper leaning against it, apparently waiting for her arrival. She thought it odd to see this cross rather than a gate.

"Congratulations!" the Gatekeeper exclaimed as she approached. "You've made it to the center of the Underworld!"

The Maiden Goddess couldn't believe it! She looked around with her arms extended to receive her baby. She had made it after all, so where was the baby she had come so far and sacrificed so much for? She couldn't wait to have that newborn in her arms. But there was no baby. All she saw was the cross and the Gatekeeper.

Finally, the Gatekeeper said, "You haven't completed your journey yet. You must cross a final threshold—the threshold between life and death." She pointed at the crucifix signaling that the Maiden Goddess would need to hang to her death!

You want to crucify me?!" The Maiden Goddess gasped, "No, I'm here to receive life, not death." The Maiden Goddess was very confused. How could death be the final threshold when she was coming for birth? This must be a mistake.

But the Gatekeeper only said, "This is the sacrifice required. You must allow your inner Maiden to die so your inner Mother can be born."

At that moment, the Maiden Goddess understood the entire journey. She understood all the sacrifices that were required to get her to this point, where she was willing to sacrifice her life with death. She was not the same Maiden from that sun-filled world. This journey had changed her—transformed her profoundly. She had become courageous and sovereign, vulnerable and trusting, embodied and supported, and she had fully embraced her inner power. Her old self must finally die because her new self is so much more equipped for the journey of motherhood.

So the Maiden Goddess, with pride and purpose, agreed to the sacrifice. She climbed up on that crucifix and allowed herself to fully and intentionally surrender to her death. And die, the goddess did.

The Final Gate of Transformation

Can you believe that we finally made it the center of the Underworld at our final gate? With the Maiden Goddess, together, we have faced fear, shame, expectations, disassociation, independence, and pain. We've sacrificed our metaphorical sword of protection, the cloak of modesty, map of direction and control, our shoes of pain prevention, our ability to walk, and the opportunity to numb ourselves from pain. In return, we've gained so much more. We now have the power of courage, the strength of vulnerability, the guidance of our inner wisdom, the presence of embodiment, the trust of Sacred Partnership, and the fortitude and endurance to face all kinds of pain—all the makings of a goddess, the qualities of a mother. But before we can finally transition into motherhood and hold our babies in our arms, we must be walk through this final gate—the Gate of Intentional Surrender.

This gate is very different than the others because instead of crossing a threshold, this time the Maiden Goddess must willingly climb up on her own crucifix and *allow* herself to die. The keyword here is "allow" for that is where sacrifice transforms into power. Should she be dragged onto the crucifix, she would become a martyr rather than a mother and her experience would become one of trauma rather than empowerment. So, the Maiden Goddess must choose for herself to allow death to wash over her. This is the ultimate sacrifice: to allow the maiden to die. And the ultimate sacrifice of life is always death. But once she surrenders to her fate, she finally crosses the threshold of motherhood and can move into divine celebration of her long and transformative journey (we'll explore this in Chapter 9).

This moment of death and surrender is tricky and often confusing when we don't understand this gate or any of the Gates of Transformation that have come before. The Maiden Goddess herself says, "I'm here to receive life, not death" so when we approach this gate, many women in labor can feel duped or unable to continue. But just like the Maiden Goddess, laboring women must accept and surrender to death to receive life. Because death is full transformation. It is the energy of one thing becoming another—a moving into a different state of being—a step toward enlightening—the next step into motherhood.

The Death of the Maiden

In our modern-day culture, we often think of death as the end of something. And in many ways, it is. When we have a baby, we can't go back to the way things were, who we were, the ideas we had, or how we lived our lives before. Everything is different, transformed, and changed. The past is over, and we have a new future to look forward to. And because of this sacrifice, we are elevated to a higher experience of ourselves and the meaning of our lives.

But another way to look at death is that it's not the end, just the end of things as we know them. Nothing really ever dies—it just transforms, changes, shifts, and moves. In the case of physical death, it's the end of the spirit in the body, but the spirit doesn't die; it transforms. In the case of the ego death, it's the end of the ego in the control chair, but the ego doesn't die, it transforms into something better. So, in the case of the death of the Maiden, the Maiden doesn't die, she simply transforms and enlightens into Mother. It's as if we change the prescription on the lens we see life through, and we get to see life a little brighter, a little clearer, and a little more enhanced. We get to see our purpose differently because our own lives mean so much to someone else—our children.

Death marks our graduation into self-mastery. When death occurs, it means that we have mastered that aspect of ourselves and that there are no more lessons to be learned at that level. And because the soul is always learning, transformation must happen, so death occurs and transforms us into something new, something more. And as something new, we can learn a whole new set of lessons from a whole new vantage point. When we climb up on our metaphorical crucifixes and allow ourselves to die, we are surrendering to our own self-mastery and saying to the world, "I'm ready to become new! I'm ready for a whole new set of lessons, challenges, emotions, and experiences as something new." This is what happens when we successfully and powerfully transition into motherhood.

However, if we don't willingly climb up on our crucifixes and die, but we still bring life into the world, we don't properly birth ourselves as mothers. When this happens, we often struggle with all the Gates of Transformation in our postpartum experience. We end up feeling resentful that we can't do whatever we want anymore, we long for the days before baby, we try to do everything on our own, we fight and resist, and overall, we hang on to our maidenhood when we should be embracing motherhood. Needless to say, this causes a lot of unnecessary emotional and psychological suffering. So, learning to surrender to this gate ensures a powerful entry into motherhood.

The Symbol of the Crucifix

So why does she have to crucify herself? Why the drama of being hung and slowly dying rather than a quick gunshot to the head? Well, the answer is ingrained deep in our human history. There is a mythic archetype expressed from the beginning of time that a messiah-like savior is hung to die on a crucifix or tree only to ascend later into heaven. From Krishna in India (1200 BC), to Quetzalcoatl of Mexico (587 BC), and 14 other characters in literature and religion including Jesus Christ of Nazareth (30

AD), it is clear that we humans resonate with and love to tell this archetypal story. Even our own goddess story is based on the ancient myth of *Inanna's Descent into the Underworld* (2112–04 BC) and is the earliest example of this archetype. We also see it in Tarot as the Hanged Man. The act of hanging is what is important here. The time, the pain, and the sacrifice are all amplified with a slow death rather than a quick one. In a quick death, there is no time to think, to speak, to talk, to choose. But to choose to hang slowly and accept the experience is the true sacrifice.

The same can be said for the transition from Maiden-to-Mother. Those last few centimeters of the cervix fully opening to allow the baby's head to birth through can feel like the longest and most drawn-out experience. This is the hanging period where we intentionally surrender to deeper and deeper death before we can resurrect as Mother Goddesses. We must surrender over our natural instincts of survival, of fight-flight-freeze, of resistance to death, and instead melt into the transformation. In many ways, we've already done this through every single gate up until this point. We've already sacrificed many times over and surrendered to many mini-deaths with each crossing of a threshold. Each Gate of Transformation has already taught us how to surrender to the final sacrifice—death. In most births we've attended, right at the transition point, the mother yells out, "I'm dying!" even if she has no idea about the Gates of Transformation. This is because, on a very real level, we know death is occurring, or at least it feels like it. That can bring up all kinds of emotions and thoughts that need to be surrendered to. So, let's look at what it actually means to surrender.

The Meaning of Surrender

"Surrender." That can be a very charged or triggering word. So can sacrifice. When we don't understand the power of sacrifice or surrender, it can make us feel victimized by the experience. When we are fighters by nature, incredibly surviving difficult life situations, surrender can feel not just like a death sentence, but like the obliteration of our souls. It can feel way too dangerous to even consider. It can also invoke feelings of failure, victimization, and trauma if we don't really understand what it means to surrender. So, let's clear up any misunderstandings.

To intentionally surrender is to *consciously* choose to give the protection and care of our minds, bodies, and spirits over to another person, place, or energy. We hand over the welfare of our own being, while still maintaining full sovereignty. We give over control to someone or something else, while still being in control of our own reactions, emotions, and thoughts.

In birth, we are asked to surrender to the wisdom of our bodies, to the soul path of our babies, to the threads of fate, and to a higher power. With each gate, we intentionally get out of our own way by walking through the Gates of Transformation so that the orchestra of miracles composed by energies beyond our control is free to dance, move, and make sweet music. When we do this, we have empowering and pleasurable births. That can be confusing if we haven't experienced it firsthand! How does empowerment come from surrender? Often, surrender is the term used when we have failed, like in a battle. In a way, this is true for birth too. When we stop battling ourselves and fly that white flag, we accept our fate, and this is the essence of intentional surrender.

This is usually the missing piece of the puzzle in most birth stories because surrender requires us to overcome fear, face shame, release control, rely on others, feel our pain, and embody vulnerability—it is the experience of all the Gates of Transformation all at once. So, if we haven't been moving through the Gates of Transformation, this ultimate act of death feels like it is too much. But even the most controlling and anal-retentive woman can get to this place if she allows herself to go through her own gates in her labor, and even the most submissive and easy-going woman can struggle at the crucifix of death if she resists her own gates in her labor. Personality has nothing to do with this process. It is all about acceptance and willingness to face our own darkness, make our own sacrifices, and climb up on our own crucifixes. If we do that, we walk away from birth with an indescribable sense of victory, empowerment, and readiness into motherhood.

What Happens When We Fight Surrender?

Because surrender is required at each gate in mini-doses as well as in the ultimate act of surrender at the final gate, when we fight surrender, we really put ourselves in a tough position. We run the risk of not moving through the gates in labor, so when we approach transition and pushing, we are just not ready to die. It is too overwhelming, and it can lead to feelings of victimization, trauma, and panic. When we haven't walked through the gates with intentional surrender, and perhaps have been dragged through, this final sacrifice feels like too much. We've often seen momas suffer from postpartum depression and psychosis from this type of experience, which is why it is so very important to learn how to surrender.

Resisting surrender can also have physical consequences. When we resist, our bodies become rigid as we are in fight-flight-freeze mode. When we are in this survival mode, we stop allowing, stop surrendering, and put our bodies in the energy of "NO." We start to send messages to our babies that it is too dangerous to be born right now and that something is wrong. Resistance always increases adrenaline. This can put a baby in distress if it's ready to go. The heart rate increases, and alarm bells go off in the hospital and within the baby. This can cause complications, stops labor, and ultimately result in unwanted interventions or even an emergency C-section.

A DOULA'S BIRTH STORY

Dani was a VBAC (vaginal birth after cesarean) mom because her first child required a C-section because he was breech. She did her research and emotional work and was determined to have a VBAC for her second child. The baby was in the right position all of her pregnancy, so when Dani went into labor, she felt confident that she was going to have a successful VBAC. As she moved into active labor, naturally, her contractions and sensations grew in intensity. Because she didn't get to labor at all in her previous birth, she was taken by surprise at the level of sensation that was coming through her uterus.

Her Gates of Transformation began to appear, but Dani was unprepared. I could see that she was fighting each gate because her body became increasingly tense and protective. She started to get leg cramps, and her jaw ached from clenching so hard. I encouraged her to soften into the sensation and to express what was going on for her emotionally, but she couldn't take her attention away from her pain. Her self-awareness turned into suffering as she begged for an epidural. The moment she did, the baby flipped in labor and became breech. Dani was devastated. How could this happen? She knew that if the baby didn't flip back, a C-section was the only way this birth was going to go. Her husband and I managed to calm her down and get her to focus on her feelings. I never got a chance to talk to her about the Gates of Transformation prenatally, because I was a late hire. But I decided to share with her what was happening on an emotional and spiritual level. She began to calm down and look relieved to have the language and framework around what was happening. Her mind could understand the gates, and that made them less terrifying. So, she faced her first two gates, the Gates of Courage and Sovereignty and the Gate of Vulnerability. She had to come to terms with the fact that her baby may be born via C-section; could she sacrifice her anxiety and plan for love and acceptance of what was happening? She surrendered and agreed to the C-section. But as soon as she did, her baby flipped back and engaged in her pelvis. It seemed like a miracle, but I knew that her baby wanted her to walk through the Gates of Transformation with intentional surrender. It took only another six hours of gate crossing, and Dani had her VBAC and her beautiful baby in her arms!"

As witnessed by Alexandria Moran

The Gates of Transformation can help us gain deeper and stronger sovereignty, but this can only be achieved through surrender, as we can see in the story above. When we fight surrender in labor, we lose our sovereignty and our vulnerability and invite in other energies to dictate the experience for us—whether that is our own emotions taking over or the agenda of someone else, let's say a doctor or nurse. This is when we can feel that our birth runs away with us and we can get stuck at certain gates, like in fear or shame. This is what we want to avoid by encouraging ourselves to lean into intentional surrender.

How Do We Surrender as a Natural Fighter?

But how do we lean in to surrender if it's just in our personality to fight? In this section, we speak to the women who have been survivors in life and have a natural inclination to fight rather than surrender. Learning that intentional surrender is the greatest act of courage, and the final initiation into motherhood can seem easier for those that have not had to fight their entire lives.

Many strong-minded women struggle with this gate because it is a matter of vulnerability. How vulnerable do we allow ourselves to be? Allowing our own death is the ultimate act of vulnerability. So, if we haven't walked through the Gate of Vulnerability (see Chapter 3), and conquered our resistance to it, it is going to be much harder to cross the threshold of death and surrender to the annihilation of the Maiden.

Understanding what triggers us when we go into fight-flight-freeze mode can be very helpful in allowing ourselves to become vulnerable. Is it an emotion, a scenario, or a feeling of being disrespected or dismissed? What makes us feel like we need to fight? And who are we fighting? Ourselves? Others? Our partners? Fate? The Divine? Doing the Integration Practices at the end of this chapter can really help unpack and understand our natural need to fight.

Often this fighting is for the survival of the self. We fear that we don't know who we are on the other side of death, so we avoid death at all costs. This works great in everyday life, but in circumstances that require a death/rebirth cycle (like in labor), this can get us stuck at the Gate of Courage and Sovereignty (see Chapter 2). By recognizing that we are fighting ourselves, we can cultivate courage as needed at the moment to embrace the unknown and lean into the sacrifice required.

At other times our resistance is rooted in a history where no one really helped or stood up for us as children. We had to learn to do everything on our own. We couldn't rely on the help of others. If this is the case, going back to the Gate of Sacred Partnership (see Chapter 6) and teaching ourselves to surrender to co-dependence can be extremely helpful at this final gate.

Perhaps our fight is more with destiny or fate than anything else? Are we fighting what is happening right now? Are we stuck at the Gate of Expectations (see Chapter 4) and just can't seem to allow things to unfold as they are? This is a very common fight when our labors look different from how we anticipated. But learning to surrender our expectations, and trust that everything is unfolding exactly as it should, teaches us how to walk through this ultimate Gate of Transformation as well.

Finally, asking ourselves what kind of message our resistance and fighting sends to the baby can be really helpful in breaking down our strong walls. If we can start to reframe our fighting as not fighting against the natural flow of birth but fighting for our baby's right to be born as they require, even if it is against our own desires, can be very healing. Are we fighting for our baby or against our baby? What if we changed our perspective and instead of fighting to save ourselves, we instead fight for a loving birth? Instead of fighting for survival, what if we fight for love, support, and peace? What if our fight were elevated to something greater than ourselves? Perhaps then we could feel more inspired to make this ultimate sacrifice.

We've also seen that when moms realize their thoughts, feelings, and beliefs directly affect their babies in labor, they tend to have a much easier time surrendering to this final sacrifice of death. We must ask ourselves, what kind of message are we sending our babies when we resist our own Maiden death? Are we telling our babies that they are welcomed or unwelcomed? Are we instilling confidence in our babies that we trust and have the courage or that we are afraid and incapable of serving them? Are we fighting to save ourselves or are we fighting for a loving birth? Do we want our babies to feel empowered and strong as they move through the birth canal, or scared and hesitant? When we realize how our own internal messaging affects our babies in labor, it can often make it much easier to just surrender, because we are doing it for someone else, not just ourselves.

Embodiment and Surrender

Another thing to consider is that embodiment is a precursor to intentional surrender. Just think about it for a moment. How can we choose to surrender to spiritual death if no one is home? The body won't allow us to. When we are not embodied, our bodies work on autopilot and behave accordingly. Our default setting as humans is "don't die." So, in labor, when we understand many deaths need to happen, our body simply won't surrender without its captain (the soul) overriding the default setting. This is why we call this gate, "Intentional Surrender." Our souls need to be steering the ship, making the calls, intentionally for this to work.

A great thing to consider when struggling with surrender is to ask, "Am I embodied? Or is my body on autopilot?" The moment we return to our bodies, we can actually choose to intentionally surrender. Without embodiment, we don't have much of a chance at moving through this Gate of Transformation.

A DOULA'S BIRTH STORY

Janet was an older first-time mom, about 41 years old when she went into labor. I was hired last minute, so I didn't get a chance to really know Janet and her backstory. The first time we met in person was at the hospital while she was in active labor. Janet was a yoga instructor and a very embodied woman. I could tell right away that she was easily surrendering to her gates throughout labor. As I learned from her partner, Janet had suffered many stillbirths and miscarriages, so she was 100 percent all-in for labor. She had waited for this experience her whole life and fully embraced everything with courage and gratitude. I was wondering to myself why she wanted me to be there since she was really doing a great job laboring and connecting to her baby and her partner.

Janet surrendered beautifully through all the gates, multiple times, and her labor was progressing quickly. We were there for about five hours, and she started wanting to push. The nurse said she could start to push if she wanted to, but it would probably be a while. So, Janet allowed her body to guide her, and she pushed when she felt the urge. But about two pushes in, I saw something shift in her eyes. I could literally see her spirit leave her body. She looked zoned out or frozen. I asked her to come back to this moment, to look into my eyes and stay present. We focused on breathing to bring her back into her body, and she came back. But a few pushes later, I could see that she left again! We used the breathing to bring her back, but I could tell that pushing was going to end up being complicated if we didn't figure out what was going on. After 30 minutes of little progression, the doctor started to talk C-section, which just brought more fear into the space.

I asked her, "What is coming up for you right now?" She said that she was afraid that the baby would be dead, like her other ones, and she wouldn't be able to survive another stillborn experience. She started to convince herself that a C-section would be better. The nurse and I reassured her that the baby had a strong heartbeat and that she was fully capable of pushing her baby out. I could see she was still fighting, resisting, and holding on to the fear. She would not surrender to her body, to the pushing or to what was actually happening. I simply said to her, "Right now, if you want, you can give your baby the gift of being fully present to receive her. You can choose to be right here with her or not. Can you choose to be fully present, not for yourself, but for your baby?"

Because she was a yoga instructor, she understood on a body level what that meant, and she immediately summoned the courage to face her fears of stillbirth for a higher purpose—to be a welcoming and embodied mother to her newborn baby girl. With this newfound motivation, she fully surrendered to her body, and her baby came popping out after only a few pushes! Janet's willingness to surrender to her fear of death made a big difference in the outcome of her labor and her connection with her new daughter. Her bravery was something I will remember forever.

As witnessed by Alexandria Moran

Knowing Your Birth Rights

One of the things we are always surprised about is the lack of understanding around simple, human birth rights. We've seen many women struggle to walk through certain gates, and especially this final gate, all because they didn't know what their rights were. And they aren't to blame. The medical community, insurance companies, and the entertainment industry really confuse and blur the lines of a woman's right to birth. Perhaps this is why the United States has one of the highest maternal and newborn death rates of any industrialized country! Women just don't know their rights and hand over their sovereignty as a result.

Learning to surrender can be so much easier when we understand the boundaries and parameters of our natural human rights. When our rights are upheld, surrender is that much easier. However, if at any time our boundaries get crossed, we can choose to step out of surrender mode, act as needed to support ourselves and to return our rights. Once we re-establish our boundaries we can then bring ourselves back into surrender mode. This is the ultimate act of sovereignty. If this feels like too much, we can ask our partners to help us return our rights so that we can focus on labor. Knowledge is power, and having the power over our own bodies allows us to feel comfortable surrendering the care of it to another.

But we need to know what those rights are! So what are our birth rights? They differ slightly from state to state, country to country, but we all have fundamental human rights that should not be forgotten just because we are in labor:

- Every person has the right to receive safe and appropriate maternity care.
- Every person has the right to maternity care that respects their fundamental human dignity.
- Every person has the right to privacy and confidentiality.
- Every person is free to make choices about their own pregnancy and childbirth, even if their caregivers do not agree with them.
- Every person has the right to equality and freedom from discrimination.

These rights are simple, but many, if not all, can be forgotten or just ignored by medical providers, staff, and even family/caregivers. These five rights are wonderful to put into the Energetic Birth Plan and to use throughout pregnancy, during labor, birth, and postpartum. We are all human and deserve the same rights as anyone else.

Being in a vulnerable space may make us worry that our rights will be taken advantage of—and this is valid. As doulas, we've seen all sorts of scenarios where this happens. This is why it is super important to have the Sacred Partner (see Chapter 6) be on the lookout for rights violations, so the laboring mom doesn't have to. When we truly believe in our basic human rights, it becomes much harder for them to be taken away during our most vulnerable time, labor. Integrating these rights into boundary work (see Chapter 3) can be incredibly healing and empowering.

How to Walk Through the Gate of Intentional Surrender

The following suggestions are great ways to intentionally surrender, not only to this final gate, but also to all the previous gates that have come before.

Walk Through All the Gates

The best way of learning how to intentionally surrender is to do the work of walking through the gates. You can start now in pregnancy and get yourself very prepared for the labor experience. Journal, share, and communicate what it is like to walk through different gates with your birth team. The more familiar you are with your own resistance, habits, and programs, the easier it will be to recognize them in labor. If your birth team understands your process, they may be able to recognize certain patterns when you can't. This can be an invaluable tool when you get stuck or confused. So share yourself. Share your process. Get vulnerable now so you can be powerful and supported in labor.

Get Vulnerable

Speaking of vulnerability, start to get really comfortable with your own. Challenge yourself to do things that take you out of your comfort zone. Spread your legs wide if that makes you feel uncomfortable. Speak your opinion if you find yourself holding back. Share your secrets if you hide your truth. Practice vulnerability as much and as often as you can. The moms who can be vulnerable often have the shortest and most empowering birth experiences!

Allow the Lessons of the Previous Gates to Guide You

This may seem obvious, but it isn't. Just because we walk through the gates doesn't mean we are going to remember what we learned or even what we gained. Communicating your experience with your birth team can help them help you to remember. When you forget your courage, your birth partner can say, "Remember when you went through that one gate, and this happened, but you did this, and that really worked for you? Do you want to try that?" Just having this kind of support with the emotional sacrifices and gates can be life-changing in labor. So, let the lessons you've learned reap the rewards and when you forget, ask your birth team to remind you!

Lean on Your Sacred Partner

We cannot surrender intentionally if we don't feel safe. Allow the work that you do through the Gate of Sacred Partnership in Chapter 6 to create a safe and sacred space where you feel 100 percent safe. Work with your Sacred Partner in pregnancy to build trust, so that even when you feel like you can't trust labor, your body, the doctors or anything else, at least you can trust and lean on this person. Your Sacred Partner can make or break this final gate by how powerfully secure they can make you feel while you labor.

Focus on Embodiment

As mentioned earlier in the chapter, this gate is impossible to work through if you're on autopilot. Becoming accustomed to embodiment is vital in facing the spiritual death of the Maiden. We highly recommend walking through the Gate of Embodiment (see Chapter 5) as many times as you can before labor so that when you are asked to climb up on your crucifix, you can do so with sovereignty and empowerment. This is the single most important state of being for walking through this gate.

INTEGRATION PRACTICES

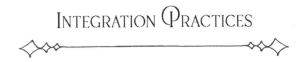

The following practices are intended to help you integrate the information of this chapter and apply it to your life now, so you can walk through this Gate of Transformation with intentional surrender and trust while in labor! Take your time going through the practices that resonate the most with you and feel free to do them as often as you'd like.

SELF-LOVE ACTIVITY: THE SPIRIT OF SURRENDER COLLAGE

Creating a collage can be a simple but powerful integration tool to help work out any kinks, blocks, or resistance to surrender. You can create a Pinterest board or do it the old-fashioned way with a poster-board, magazines, and a glue stick. If you are doing it the old-fashioned way, get a poster-board and draw a line down the middle. On the left-hand side write, "The Energy of My Resistance" and on the right-hand side write, "The Energy of My Surrender." If you are doing a Pinterest board, make two different boards for each state of being. Then start to collect images from magazines and/or the Internet that represent these two energies. When you are done pasting and organizing your chosen images, take a look at the difference visually. What do you notice? If you'd like, share with your birth team and help them remind you of this energy difference when you are in the throes of resistance. You can even bring the board to your birth for a healthy reminder.

SELF-LOVE ACTIVITY: SAYING YES FOR A DAY

Sometimes when we struggle to surrender, we find ourselves getting stuck in a NO mentality. We say "no" to people, places, things, and even to ourselves almost out of habit and self-preservation. But surrender is the opposite of self-preservation. In this exercise, you will not be allowed to say "no" to anyone or anything for a whole day. Instead, you must practice surrendering to the things you don't want to do and the effort you don't want to make. As you start to say "yes" more throughout your day, you may find much more happiness and expansion of the heart through this simple self-love act. It is important to note that this exercise doesn't trump boundary violations, criminal activity, or anything dangerous, so make sure to use common sense and good safety throughout the day. You can journal your experience at the end.

INNER EXPLORATION JOURNAL PROMPTS

The following journal prompts are for you to explore and uncover the different challenges of this gate. The practice of journaling can be deeply healing and enlightening, so we encourage you to spend some time reading over the prompts to see which ones resonate with you. Look back at these often. You might notice that different journal prompts resonate at different times.

Resistance

- What emotions do I dislike experiencing? What emotions do I typically resist?
- What emotions are annoying to deal with, but which I usually can?

- What emotions do I dare not touch with a 20-foot stick?
- How can I become better at surrendering my resistance?
- How do I do when things don't go my way? How does it make me feel? Which gates are still difficult for me after working through this book?

Surrendering

- What is my natural response to pain or trauma? Fight? Flight? or Freeze?
- What feelings come up when I think about the word surrender?
- Am I a natural fighter? If so, what do I find myself fighting the most? Myself? Fate? Circumstance?
- What do I need to feel safe to surrender?
- In what circumstances am I not great at surrendering?
- In what circumstances am I really great at surrendering?

GODDESS RITUAL: A FUNERAL FOR THE MAIDEN

Rituals are a powerful way to anchor and fully accept transitions. One of the best ways to really accept the death of the Maiden is to create a funerary ritual for your Maiden-self. Funerals give us closure and create a space to grieve our loss. Doing this consciously and with intention for our Maiden-selves can be a great thing to do before labor starts and can give us the necessary closure needed to climb up on our crucifixes and allow the Maiden-selves to fully die.

Ideas for Funerary Practices

- Write a letter to your Maiden-self, thanking her and expressing what you will miss about her.
- Write a eulogy for your Maiden-self.
- Bury a symbolic item (e.g., crystal, feather, chicken bones, etc.) that represents your Maiden-self. The act of digging a grave and burying the past can be very cathartic.
- Create a piece of art to commemorate her life and death.

GODDESS RITUAL: CREATE A DEATH ALTAR

You have already created a birth altar to focus your intentions for your pregnancy and labor. It's now time to create a death altar for our Maiden-self. If you recall, an altar is a special space that you set aside as a sacred spot in your home to hold your intention and return to in uncertainty. You can place this altar next to your birth altar as a reminder to the ultimate sacrifice of the Maiden death.

What You Need:

- Small flat space to place items
- Objects, crystals, candles, images or anything that symbolizes your own Maiden death

What to Do:

Take some time for yourself to meditate on the meaning of your Maiden death and collect objects that symbolize the end of the era. You might choose to use old photos, mementos, crystals, or candles as a way of honoring the end of your maidenhood. You might also choose to combine this ritual with the funerary ritual given above.

GODDESS RITUAL: MAIDEN-TO-MOTHER AFFIRMATION

Say the following affirmation as often as you like aloud, quietly or as a mantra over and over again as you transition from Maiden-to-Mother. Place your hands over your crown chakra and say: *"I intentionally surrender to the death of my old, Maiden-self as I birth the next version of myself. I am ready to be Mother."*

THRESHOLD MEDITATION

In this meditation, you'll go on a short journey through this gate to allow your Maiden-self to die. This is a great meditation to practice for this ultimate sacrifice and will bring up a lot of feelings and hidden understandings. This practice can be done after each journal prompt or daily until you feel complete in your transition. It is also a great meditation for labor when moments of resistance show up or right before transition. Visit www.laborlikeagoddess.com to download it.

Final Thoughts

The strength, courage, and trust it takes to intentionally surrender are life-changing. Now that you have this skill and information, it will be available to use throughout your everyday life. When you started on your journey into your emotional Underworld through the Gates of Transformation, the idea of complete surrender seemed daunting, but the sacrifice of Motherhood isn't complete without it. You've become a goddess through this gate and have fully moved into your Mother-self! Take these lessons and this journey into your parenting and your daily life with your family.

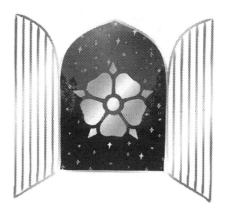

CHAPTER IX

MOTHERHOOD, A DIVINE INITIATION

POSTPARTUM LIKE A GODDESS

Breathe. You're going to be okay. Breathe and remember that you've been in this place before. You've been this uncomfortable and anxious and scared, and you've survived. Breathe and know that you can survive this too.

—*Daniell Koepke*

$\mathcal{B}$ut, then in a blink of an eye, the Maiden Goddess found herself gasping for air. She was back in her sun-filled world, reborn, with a newborn baby in her arms, and her beloved was holding them both.

The Moon had kept her promise. She was now a mother and was gazing upon the most precious child she had ever seen. All the fear, all the shame, all the control, all the pain, all the indignity, all the sacrifice suddenly became so worth it, and she finally could see that the greatest rewards come from the greatest sacrifices.

It was all worth it. . . a thousand times over! She was flooded with joy, love, and so much gratitude. She was exhausted but had never felt more powerful in her entire life. "Thank you, Moon," she uttered, feeling a deep sense of power, pleasure, and pride in her own fortitude and transformation. She was now a mother.

Divine Celebration

CONGRATULATIONS, MAMA!!! WOOOOOHOOOOOO!!! YOU MADE IT! What a journey we've been on together! You've proven your courage, your strength of character, your willingness to sacrifice, and your power to transform the old into the new. You are a true Mother Goddess, and now you get to bask in the glory of all your hard work—your baby is finally here. The Moon and the Underworld have kept their promise and rewarded you with the greatest gift. Was it worth it? Heck yes! This is a time of great celebration, deep honoring and reverence for this miracle. So pop those bottles and celebrate! You deserve it.

The following chapter isn't a gate of transformation like all the rest, but instead contains tips, tricks, and advice to support you during this initial postpartum phase, because the truth is, you are about to embark on a whole other journey into early motherhood. But for now, soak up the energy of your amazing accomplishment and transformation.

This is a time of reverence and deep bows to you, Mother Goddess, and it is time to let yourself receive them. One rather trendy and popular way to honor your transition is with a "push gift." This is great for moms whose love language is gifts. (If you haven't read *The Five Love Languages* by Gary Chapman, we highly recommend it now that you are a mom and you get to learn the love language of your new family member.) This gift is best given by the life partner as a way to recognize and honor your amazing journey—although you can also give one to yourself. If your love language is something different, such as "acts of service," have your life partner give a more fitting gift. This way, it feels personal and tailored to your own love language.

It's also a great idea to honor your life partner's transition into parenthood too if you have one, to mark the huge shift that has occurred and honor their role as a co-parent. These gifts and acts of acknowledgment go a long way in accepting our births just as they are. You'll find more ways of honoring this transition in our Integration Practices at the end of this chapter.

The Gates of Integration

Now that you have successfully completed the *Labor Like a Goddess* journey, you are now embarking on a whole different one: *Postpartum Like a Goddess*! But instead of Gates of Transformation, this journey will mean traversing the Gates of Integration. The next year of your life will be all about integrating this huge shift from Maiden-to-Mother and all the feelings, thoughts, and experiences that come with this huge integration. In a future book, we will break down these gates one by one, but we wanted to leave you with a few tips and offerings to help you better understand this next very powerful phase of life.

The Power of Accepting Our Births

Acceptance is the greatest gift we can give ourselves after this long, hard, and exhausting journey. For all the reasons we've already explored (including the belief that baby needs to be born a certain way for their own karmic and soul journey), accepting our births, everything that transpired, how we reacted, and how we felt is a big part of setting ourselves up for a positive postpartum experience. This is one of the first Gates of Integration that happens on the postpartum journey—allowing ourselves to find full acceptance of our birth experience, no matter what happened.

Usually right when we give birth, we are so overcome with joy that we only remember the empowering and positive aspects of the labor. We highly recommend doing a video recording of yourself telling your labor and delivery story, so you always have that to reflect on later in postpartum. This is a useful tool if you find yourself starting to feel dissatisfied with your birth experience in the coming weeks or even months afterward. If that happens, just know that working through dissatisfaction is part of the postpartum journey and going through the Gates of Integration.

Many women can find themselves feeling dissatisfied with their birth even if they didn't have a typical "traumatic birth" or even if they felt really good about their births at first, but over time, started to second-guess everything. Having a homemade video of the joy, the moment, and the story of the birth can be incredibly helpful during this very hormonal time when doubt and frustration creep in. Just know that feeling this way is absolutely normal and a huge part of walking through the postpartum Gates of Integration.

Getting Verbal Validation

It is so important to our mental health and acceptance of our birth experience to be able to receive verbal validation for what an amazing thing we have just accomplished. Allow yourself to be showered with praise, especially from your Sacred Partner (see Chapter 6) who witnessed your labor. This praise is a great way to anchor the positivity of the experience. Validation is an important part of self-esteem, and as new mothers, we are so open, so vulnerable, and so impressionable, that having positive, empowering, and uplifting words can deeply heal any dissatisfaction or lingering negative emotions.

When you as a mother feel validated, it translates to your baby, and they begin to develop positive self-esteem. The more love and praise you allow yourself to receive will actually bring greater love and validation to your baby. In our experience, this can help to curtail all kinds of early newborn problems like colic or issues with breastfeeding. So, let yourself be showered with love so both you and your baby can receive the benefits.

When We Aren't Able to Celebrate

What happens when we find ourselves unable to celebrate this journey—either due to postpartum depression, trauma, or loss? Even if we don't have a traumatic birth experience, it can sometimes be hard emotionally to celebrate the accomplishment of entering motherhood. If you find yourself in this position, please know that you are not alone. So many women are going through what you are going through. Baby blues are a natural part of "coming down" from pregnancy and the highs of the labor hormones, and every mom gets at least a little bit of the blues. Up to 80 percent of moms report frequent and prolonged crying, feelings of anxiousness, sadness, irritability, depression, panic, frustration, worry, deep vulnerability, and feelings of hopelessness[8]. Even sleep, appetite, and concentration are affected. After all, it is also a time of deep grief for the death of the Maiden and redefinition of our identities.

This is the beginning of the integration period of motherhood—feeling so much love for the baby yet so much loss for ourselves. This mixed bag of emotions can often be overwhelming, confusing, and alienating to a new mom. If you feel the baby blues, know that's okay, and that's normal. This is where self-love, community, and connection with other moms going through the same blues can be a really powerful way to feel better, or at least not alone in it.

Sometimes baby blues can turn into something more intense, especially if there's been some kind of recent trauma or very intense birth experience. Up to 6 percent of moms experience PTSD in early motherhood, and this is where mom feels strongly that her life and her baby's life are in danger or at risk[9]. Reaching out, asking for help, and connecting with a professional will help you move through this very curable and very treatable experience. If you find yourself going deeper than baby blues, know that help is available and effective. Check out our Recommended Resources at the back of this book for more information.

No matter the intensity of feeling you experience—whether baby blues or something more—remember your Gates of Transformation. You may have to face some shames, fears, and expectations, and the exercises in this book can help you move through them. And remember that the Divine Masculine energy can be a saving grace during this period of integration. Let yourself share with your partner, your doula, or whoever holds the Divine Masculine space for you what is really going on in your space. Empower yourself by joining a support group or working with a professional healer or therapist. It is so important to feel supported as a new mom, so ask for help as soon as you recognize you may need it. This takes a level of courage and vulnerability that you've already learned in your labor experience, so integrate that wisdom here and now for you, your baby, and your family.

Nine Months In–Nine Months Out

For the past nine months or so, you have been in a prolonged state of transition—growing, changing, but mostly preparing for this moment, the moment you can now call yourself Mother. Throughout this book, you have been guided to this exact moment. Rejoice in your accomplishment! Because a new journey is about to begin.

There is a phrase that many like to reference when describing the first part of motherhood: the fourth trimester. This term was created to describe the first three months after your baby is born as a continuation of the pregnancy period. Coincidentally, this is also the length of time it takes for a newborn to fully adjust to being outside of the womb. For animals, newborns are fairly self-sufficient at birth or shortly after. Human babies, on the other hand, take years to fully develop the skills to fend for themselves. Scientists claim that this is due to our advanced brain development. Our brain must grow over time outside of the womb. This is most critical during the first three months after birth and this is why it is really important to learn how to prepare for this period.

Just like your newborn needs time to adjust to the world, you need time to adjust to becoming a mother. The concept of *nine months in-nine months* out is a fairly new idea and describes how it takes a woman about nine months to fully heal and integrate into motherhood. Our bodies are amazing—we heal surprisingly quickly after pregnancy and birth—but that's just the beginning. The immense amount of internal healing, and integration for the changes that just occurred, takes time. Our cervix might heal completely in about six weeks, but our whole body and mind take months, if not years.

The idea of *nine months in-nine months out* is to normalize this concept, to allow women and society to understand that it takes time for the healing process, and it allows women and their families to learn how to become parents, caregivers, and supporters of the new motherhood journey. Understanding this will not only normalize how postpartum usually unfolds, but also equalize the roles of men, women, and society in the full birth experience.

Looking back at the Goddess journey, we can now truly understand the enormous feat it was. Walking through each Gate of Transformation, the Maiden Goddess gained wisdom that not only helped during pregnancy and labor but will also prove useful in motherhood. Her goal was simple: to become a mother. But, now that this goal has been fulfilled, what comes next? How can the Maiden Goddess succeed in motherhood? In parenting? The answer: She must utilize the knowledge and skills she gained from each of the Gates of Transformation and apply them in her everyday life with her child. And we must do so as well.

Diving Deep into Motherhood

Throughout the fourth trimester and into the first full year of motherhood, every day, week, and the month are full of immense change. Starting from week one, you are exhausted from labor—rightfully so. Your body immediately starts to heal. Your breast milk starts to come in, and you become a new vessel—a body that can nourish your baby. During pregnancy, you were nourishing your baby without knowing it. Your body took over. The placenta was formed, and your baby ate whenever they wanted to. The only thing you needed to worry about was feeding yourself. Now nourishment is in your hands.

This can be really jarring for many women, your beautiful little baby comes out ready to latch and suckle, but as modern women, we often have no idea how to breastfeed. There are a few instinctual actions that women will have, such as putting their baby on to their tummy or breast and guiding their baby's head toward their nipples. Some women have the urge to hand express their milk, but overall women only know their baby must be fed. This is all in the first moments of motherhood, a completely new experience for a first-time mother. Imagine all the other wild new things that you will go through in the first few months! This is where the wisdom and skills you learned from the Gates of Transformation can help you.

There are two ways that the Gates of Transformation will come up during the first year of motherhood: on a large scale by *being a mother,* and on a smaller one in the *decisions you make.* Understanding that the gates aren't linear, we can see how they might not flow the same way as they may have when you were preparing for labor. In fact, preparing for motherhood is the reverse—a backward spiraling. The postpartum journey starts at the culmination of childbirth, a moment of complete intentional surrender and then proceeds to work backward through the gates. On a grand scale, motherhood's gates flow from surrendering to the birth of your baby to embodiment by being in the moment with your newborn, to sharing this new experience with your partner, to feeling the pain of childbirth after the flush of hormones leave your body, to expecting to just know how to be a mother, to the shame of not knowing, and then finally to the fear of "can I even do this?" The Gates of Transformation during the first few days of motherhood show how we immediately start a new journey of self-mastery. But as you know, the gates can and will pop up when they are triggered and the flow of the gates will change for every different circumstance.

Another example of how the gates will appear during the first few weeks of motherhood is if you choose to breastfeed—this topic brings up every single gate for women:

- *The fear* (Gate of Courage and Sovereignty) of not being able to do it or not having enough milk;
- *The shame* (Gate of Vulnerability) around breast exposure, or if you even want to breastfeed or not;
- *The expectations* of ease (Gate of Expectations) that breastfeeding should come naturally and easy, when in fact it feels like you need a Ph.D. to get it right;

- *The embodying of* your decisions (Gate of Embodiment) whether to continue to breastfeed, supplement, bottle feed, or any other variation of nurturing;
- The asking for *help* (Gate of Sacred Partnership) *from a partner* or lactation consultant to get you through the day;
- *The pain of suckling* (Gate of Fortitude), of raw nipples and of bad latches;
- *The surrendering* (Gate of Intentional Surrender) to however you need or decide to nourish your baby.

This is just one of many examples of how the gates can help you navigate the first few weeks of motherhood and beyond. There are thousands of little decisions you make as a mother, each of those decisions can trigger a gate, and we hope that you will call upon your wisdom and experience with the Gates of Transformation to face each gate with courage and power.

A MOTHER'S STORY

Brooke just had her first baby; She was also the first in her family and of her friends to have a baby in many years, and also the first of her friends. Brooke didn't have many people around her with recent knowledge of childbirth and newborn life, which led her to become an expert on the topic. She took every class she could, hired a doula, and ended up becoming a doula herself. She was fascinated with the idea of birth and motherhood. The one thing Brooke didn't take into account was a personal experience. After Brooke gave birth to her baby girl (in which she walked through the gates beautifully) and had a powerful all-natural birth, she headed home from the hospital, ready to embrace all that was motherhood.

On their first night home, her baby started to cluster feed, which is normal and helps mothers produce more milk. After six hours of almost nonstop feeding, Brooke's nipples were raw and bloody and she was in severe pain. She knew something wasn't right. Brooke was scared that her baby wasn't getting enough milk or that her latch wasn't right. She started to panic— it was the middle of the night, and she knew she wouldn't be able to reach her lactation consultant. At that moment she didn't know what to do. Her baby girl had been screaming for over an hour. This wasn't how she thought the first few days of motherhood would be. She knew it was going to be hard, but this felt like torture.

As she sat in front of her crying baby, Brooke broke down. She didn't know what to do. Brooke had planned on exclusively breastfeeding and didn't want to use formula at all. But in that moment, Brooke knew that her baby needed something. She was in too much pain to pump or hand express, she tried and knew she couldn't. Then she remembered that she had received a sample of formula. Brooke decided right there that she would give her daughter 2oz of formula.

After the baby finished her bottle, she immediately fell asleep. Brooke was so relieved that her baby was content and that her breasts were able to rest and heal. The next morning Brooke woke up with a huge sense of shame. What had she done? She had gone against her plan, and made a decision that didn't align with how she expected she would mother. Crying to her lactation consultant, she turned to Brooke and said, "Your baby is happy today, your nipples were able to heal; there is nothing to be ashamed of. You made the right decision at the moment for your baby and yourself." This validation was the jumpstart of Brooke walking through her first gate as a mother facing her shame.

As told by Brooke to Lauren Mahana

Motherhood is a series of never-ending decisions, and these decisions are not yours; they are meant for another, your baby. It is difficult to know if you are making the right choice in any given moment, and with that comes the fear and shame of making a mistake. That is why Brooke was so distraught after the formula feeding. Her shame didn't come from feeding her daughter formula, it came from not sticking with her original decision. After walking through the Gate of Vulnerability and the Gate of Expectations, Brooke came to terms with her decision. Motherhood is a series of never-ending decisions and being flexible when those decisions need to change.

Baby's Past-Lives Processing

Now that we have explored your integration into motherhood, let's dive a little deeper into how your baby is processing life— not just on the physical level, but on a soul level. The idea that the soul chooses when, where, and how it will be born is something that is discussed throughout this book. We explore the idea that every soul picks their parents based on their karmic debt or cosmic path. If we believe that this is occurring, then there must be a period when this soul must also learn how to become one with this new life.

Acknowledging that your baby is also in a state of emotional transition allows you to help your baby during this time. Your baby is still processing this event, and you have a wonderful opportunity to manifest an optimal environment for your baby to settle into their new surroundings.

One way you can help achieve this goal is to follow your baby's lead, especially in the first few weeks when you both are learning how to be in your new roles: you as a mother and baby as a newborn human. You can do this by feeding on demand, holding your baby when they need to be held, keeping your home dark and quiet, and keeping your baby close to you (for example, in the same room when they're napping or sleeping as a way to guard against SIDS). This can be hard if you have other children or pets, but you can create a sanctuary space where you and the baby can rest and recharge throughout the day.

Another way is through mindfulness, intentionally thinking about how your baby is processing their past lives. Hold peaceful thoughts in your mind about how grateful you are that they choose you as their mother. Honor their spirit journey by doing simple rituals, like creating a baby album (physical or digital), or hosting a gathering of family and friends to welcome your baby into their lives. These are all ways you can honor the soul that has chosen you and your family.

A MOTHER'S STORY

This is a quick story about how Sarah found peace with motherhood. A few months into postpartum life, Sarah started to feel like a mother. Focusing on making sure her baby was taken care of, Sarah had a daily routine of feeding, changing, bathing, and playtime for her newborn, and felt a sense of accomplishment in that she was succeeding.

But one morning Sarah lifted her armpit, and oh my goddess did she stink! Sarah realized that it had been over a week since she had showered. She had been too busy to even notice. Just that small whiff of B.O. had her spiraling. It triggered gates that she thought were mastered, fear of being a dirty person and shame that she had let herself go. While immersed in the downward emotional spiral, Sarah jumped into the shower. Spending just a few minutes cleaning her body, she realized that she needed to find a balance. Sarah knew she was a good mother, her baby was happy and healthy. But she had forgotten that she also needed to take care of herself.

Knowing that she needed help remembering this, Sarah asked her husband to remind her every day at 11 a.m. to take a shower. No matter what was happening (if it was a "normal" day), she would stop what she was doing and take a shower. Of course, she would continue feeding or playtime, but the reminder and routine of showering near the 11 a.m. mark was just a moment in the day that Sarah could focus on herself. Even if it was a five-minute-long shower, she knew that she was creating a space for herself.

As told by Sarah to Lauren Mahana

In this short, simple story, Sarah realizes that motherhood is not only about caregiving to your newborn, but it's also about finding the space to care about yourself. That is the true essence of integration, allowing yourself to both give and receive, even if it's a short shower or a quick bite to eat. The following Integration Practices can help you find this internal balance for yourself and ease your integration into motherhood.

How to Walk Through Early Motherhood

Before you became a mother, self-care was probably something that was part of your normal routine. It is a big part of learning Maiden life lessons—something you may have cultivated over time to comfort and care for your physical and emotional bodies. For some, that might mean carving out a spa day once a week. For others, it's daily meditation and yoga classes or heading to the mall for a day of shopping. As long as you are healthy, there isn't a right or wrong way to self-care. But once you become a mother, your priorities change. You suddenly stop focusing only on yourself and start to focus on your baby, and in a completely different way from how you would care for any other loved one. Having a newborn is all-encompassing. You are immersed in only their needs and may not feel as though you have the time or space to take care of yourself. You might even forget your old self-care habits and dismiss them as frivolous, but they aren't. Self-care is the key to successfully integrating into motherhood. You can only take care of others if you first take care of yourself. You must allow for space for a new self-care practice. And, yes it will be different. It might not be elaborate or adventurous, but it will feed your soul in the same way.

To walk through and integrate early motherhood, creating a new self-care routine for yourself as a mother is crucial. Know that it will grow and change, so don't worry if it all seems so simple now.

Create a Routine

When you have a structure to your day, you will be able to carve out time to focus on yourself. Creating structure in the first few weeks of motherhood can feel overwhelming. But as you get into your groove and learn about your baby more and more each day, you will find that you can start to create benchmarks throughout the day. Just make sure you are carving some time for basic daily hygiene for yourself with those benchmarks.

Ask for Help

This is a big one! Remember all your training through the Gate of Sacred Partnership and draw upon those skills in motherhood. Ask a family member or friend, or hire a doula to help you. This could be as simple as making you a few meals, cleaning your home, or holding the baby when you just need a break. Help is necessary when you have a newborn. Call upon your tribal roots and reach out. We promise you will feel less overwhelmed when you have support.

Nourishment

Make sure you are eating and drinking water. It seems simple and obvious, but it is really easy to end up snacking on junk food rather than eating nutritious meals while you bounce between breastfeeding, changing diapers, and comforting or playing with your newborn. Basic nutrition can seem like one of the hardest things to accomplish during the fourth trimester. Put mealtime in your routine and make drinking water a priority. Second-time moms know that they must always grab a glass of water or healthy snack before sitting down to breastfeed. Eating when baby eats is a great way to not only ensure you are making time for your nutrition, but also to keep up your breast milk supply. Even if you are formula feeding, you are still feeding throughout the night, which can be exhausting.

Daily Hygiene

This is different for everyone, the bar for personal hygiene can range from needing to shower and wash your hair twice a day to once a week. Whatever it means to you, spend a moment and think of your Maiden hygiene routine. Did you shower every day and wash your hair once a week? Did you shower every other day? Think about how you felt the most comfortable, and then apply that same mentality to your new life. If you took a shower once a day, then continue to do so. This will help you find a balance and feel self-love in motherhood.

Community

It doesn't matter if you are an extrovert or introvert; finding a community that will support you during this time in crucial to your success in early motherhood. New mom groups, breastfeeding groups, parenting groups, music classes, social media groups, old friends, or new friends are all great ways of finding others who are going through the same thing as you—especially other mothers who have babies of similar ages. This is really important to processing the new and surprising emotions and experiences that pop up in early motherhood. Sharing the crazy experience can make you feel more at ease and comfortable with your own integration.

Now that you have a deep understanding of the importance of integrating into motherhood, let's explore different ways you can help this process. Integration isn't something that just happens. You must add small pieces of your new identity into your life over time. Some pieces might align quicker than others, but this is a process that ebbs and flows. There are no expectations with integration, just small victories.

Integration Practices

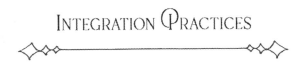

The following practices are intended to help you integrate the information of this chapter and apply it to your life now, so you can begin to walk through the Gates of Integration with empowerment! Take your time going through the practices that resonate the most with you and feel free to do them as often as you'd like.

Self-Love Activity: Celebrate!!!

This has been an incredible journey of transformation, and now is the time to celebrate. Celebration can be one of the most powerful tools to integrate the motherhood experience. Give yourself as many big and little celebrations that feel right for you and your family. Some ideas include:

- Purchase push gifts.

- Have a friend host a "Sip and See" party to introduce the baby to family and friends.
- Hermit yourself with your new little family for a few days or weeks.
- Eat celebratory foods.
- Share your news on social media.
- Indulge in every moment with your new little one.
- Take sitz baths full of aromatic and healing herbs.
- Do a new family photoshoot.
- Start a baby book to document "firsts."
- Have a belly-binding ceremony to "close" the door on pregnancy.
- Ask for blessings from family and friends.

SELF-LOVE ACTIVITY: WRITE OR RECORD A MESSAGE TO YOUR FUTURE SELF

Right after having a baby, your energy will be so full of love, hope, and excitement. This is a great time to record or write down all your feelings and experiences to remind your future self of this exact moment of early motherhood. You can also include the birth story from your eyes so your child can know all the details when they are older. This is a great tool to help your future self remember the joy, innocence, and vulnerable power of motherhood during this time, so that when things get rough—and they will—these memories can pull you through. Bonus if you have your Sacred Partner (see Chapter 6) also record a statement of the birth through their eyes.

INNER EXPLORATION JOURNAL PROMPTS

The following journal prompts are for you to explore and uncover the different challenges of this gate. The practice of journaling can be deeply healing and enlightening, so we encourage you to spend some time reading over the prompts to see which ones resonate with you. Look back at these often as you might notice that certain journal prompts resonate at different times.

Birth Processing

- How would I describe my birth experience?
- What went great during my birth?
- What was difficult? How did I handle it? How do I feel about that?
- Who or what surprised me in a good way during labor?
- Who or what was disappointing?
- Which Gates of Transformation did I have to go through during labor? What was that like for me?
- Were there any gates that I resisted and need to still work through?
- How embodied was I during birth?
- What were the sacrifices I had to make?
- What were the rewards I gained?
- What emotions have been hard for me to accept?
- Have I been able to celebrate my birth, if so, what did I do? If not, what is stopping me?

Early Motherhood

- What does integration look like to me?
- What feelings and emotions have been popping up during the first few weeks of motherhood?
- How does it feel to be a mother?
- Do I feel balanced?
- Am I feeling overwhelmed or anxious? What makes these feelings more heightened?
- What is the most difficult thing so far in motherhood?
- What are the best things so far?
- What do I struggle with daily? How can I bring more ease to my routine?
- What part of self-care do I need to balance?
- How can I bring more support to my world? Who can I reach out to?
- Which Gates of Transformation have I struggled with during the first few weeks?
- Which Gates of Transformation have been successful?

- Have I allowed others to help in my integration? If not, what is holding me back from asking for help?

GODDESS RITUAL: TRANSFORM YOUR BIRTH ALTAR INTO A MOTHERHOOD ALTAR

Returning to the birth altar you created back in Chapter 1, this ritual will be a physical transformation of your birth altar into a motherhood altar. A motherhood altar is meant to be a special place for you when life with your little one gets hard, overwhelming, or frustrating. It's a place to honor your personal sacrifices and a space of respite, even for just a few minutes. Place your altar somewhere you can go visit in privacy, away from your children, as you need it.

What You Need:

- Your birth altar from pregnancy
- New objects, crystals, candles, or images for your motherhood altar

What to Do:

Take a moment and thank your birth altar. Remove all objects and cleanse them with water or smoke—whatever calls to you. Look at all the items that were on your birth altar and keep any that resonate with your new mother energy. Add new items that represent the kind of mother you want to be. It's a great idea to include a picture of your children. You can also use crystals for strength, love, nurturing, etc., or other symbols that represent Mother Goddesses like Demeter, Hera, or your own mother. Place your items on your birth altar in an order that speaks to you or follow traditional altar rules. Do what feels best. When you are done, set some mother intentions for yourself. Seal the magic with the following prayer:

"Mother Goddess, you have walked with me throughout my pregnancy. Now I humbly ask you to help guide me through motherhood. The strength, love, and wisdom you hold is a precious gift. I give thanks to all that you offer. Mother Goddess, I honor you and myself with this altar."

Return to your altar as often as you like to refresh your energy and connect with your intentions.

GODDESS RITUAL: MOTHER AFFIRMATION

Say the following affirmation as often as you like aloud, quietly or as a mantra over and over again as you integrate into motherhood. Place one hand on your heart and one hand on your womb and say: *It is important and good to nourish not only my baby, but also myself. I honor my Mother body through good nutrition, self-care, compassion, and moments of silence.*

THRESHOLD MEDITATION

In this meditation, you'll go on short journey to integrate all the thresholds you have already walked through and allow all your emotions, thoughts, and feelings to arise, be witnessed and released. This meditation is about accepting your birth and everything that happened with love, compassion and reverence. This is a perfect meditation to do while you're breastfeeding or while your baby is resting to help find your center and give yourself some energetic love. Visit www.laborlikeagoddess.com to download it.

Final Thoughts

We are so proud of this amazing journey you've accomplished! This is truly a time of positive and divine celebration. We hope you take the time and make an effort to really pause, enjoy, and celebrate how far you have come. The first few weeks after your baby is born will feel euphoric and challenging all at the same time. It's a whirlwind of emotions, exhaustion, and adjustment to a new postpartum body, baby, relationship, and spiritual understanding. Remember, it takes nine months to fully integrate this experience, so give yourself the time, space, and compassion necessary to make these next nine months satisfying. Allow yourself to fully surrender to the embodiment of motherhood because it will fly by faster than you can say, "Labor Like a Goddess."

Conclusion

The end is just the beginning.

—*T.S. Eliot*

Hopefully, by now, you recognize how your pregnancy and labor can be your own unique call to adventure into the Underworld of your being and into the greatest sacrifice of your life—motherhood. As women braving this journey and making the small sacrifices along the way, we receive, at the end of it all, one of the most powerful gifts a woman could receive in her lifetime—a deep and expansive connection to ourselves, our babies and the Divine. This all-encompassing and life-changing reward is something that we will take with us for the rest of our lives. After all, motherhood isn't something we do, but something we embody—forever.

We hope that this book and its Divine wisdom have helped guide you, inspire you and motivate you to walk through your own Gates of Transformation so you may *Labor Like A Goddess* in your birth and in your life. As you transform yourself from Maiden-to-Mother may you remember the story of the Maiden Goddess and her journey through the challenges of fear, shame, control, trust, staying present, perseverance, and acceptance as a touchstone of hope and motivation during moments of doubt or despair. May the lessons of courage, sovereignty, inner truth, and intentional surrender live in your heart as you move through postpartum and beyond. Many blessings, Mother.

Appendix I

Energetic Birth Plan Sample

The following sample is based on Alexandria Moran's Energetic Birth Plan at 20 weeks

ALEX'S ENERGETIC BIRTH PLAN

MY ENERGETIC INTENTIONS FOR MY BIRTH·	THE CIRCUMSTANCES I PREFER AND/OR WANT TO HAPPEN·	ENERGY AND EMOTIONAL EXPERIENCE I NEED·	MY WORST-CASE SCENARIOS OR SITUATIONS THAT COULD HAPPEN·	SHOULD THE WORST HAPPEN, WHAT I CAN DO TO UPHOLD MY INTENTION·
To allow and trust my baby boy to have his own timing.	Natural labor- no induction	I need intimacy and a sense of trust between me and baby.	The doctor requires that I be induced before baby is ready to come. Talk of too big a baby or other medical issue.	I can take time to connect with baby and talk to the baby... tell him what is happening. Ask him to come sooner. Trust what I hear.
For both me and my baby to feel clear headed and connected throughout labor.	Unmedicated birth without any drugs or epidural medications.	I need connection, intuition, body wisdom, purpose and love.	Failure to progress or contractions slow and I require pitocin or a c-section.	I can walk through the gate of Intentional Surrender and trust and accept that I need some medical help as part of this baby's birth plan.
To feel empowered and womanly in my birth. To feel supported by those that I love.	Vaginal birth without forceps, vacuum or episiotomy. I prefer my husband and doula to be by my side the whole time.	I need to feel a sense of accomplishment, pride, power, success and victory all while feeling safe, loved and secure.	I have to have a c-section or other intervention during pushing. I am alone with strangers.	I can choose to accept and surrender to the death of my expectations and trust that baby is in divine hands. I can choose to trust the strangers and be fully present for myself.

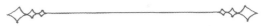
RECURRING WORDS OF INTENTION:

Trust, power, empowerment, support, connection, surrender, love

REFLECTIONS:

After writing this energetic birth plan at 20 weeks, I realized that my primary intention for my birth is to feel connected to my baby and trust that whatever happens is meant to happen. As a control freak, I found myself having to walk through so many gates, even just writing this. I notice I'm deeply afraid of being victimized by the medical community, even though I am an experienced doula. I am deeply aware of just how vulnerable I feel being pregnant and how I must truly surrender to the Gate of Expectations. A part of me feels that because I am so knowledgeable about birth that I can control my "perfect" birth experience. After writing this, I realize how much surrender actually still needs to happen. I also am starting to see how my need to "control" my birth is actually interfering with my connection to my baby—which is the one thing I really really want and mention many times throughout this plan.

STATEMENT OF COMMITMENT

I commit to walking through the Gate of Expectations and the Gate of Intentional Surrender to improve my ability to trust, connect and accept any and all outcomes to my birth experience with love, gratitude and peace for myself and my baby boy.

ENERGETIC BIRTH INTENTION

I intend to bring the energy of peace, surrender, openness, and love to my birth space with full trust, honor, and acceptance of everything and anything that happens or needs to happen to safely birth my baby boy.

Appendix II

Sacred Contract Sample

The following contract is based on the one drawn up by Alexandria Moran and husband, Murray in readiness for labor.

ALEX'S SACRED PARTNERSHIP CONTRACT

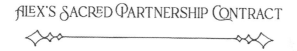

I, Alexandria Moran, enter into Sacred Partnership with husband Murray Moran for the purpose of, together, birthing a baby into the world in the winter of 2019/2020 with love, trust, peace, and safety. For the duration of this pregnancy, throughout labor, delivery, and into the first three months of postpartum, I enter into these vows:

· I promise to allow myself to be the full embodiment of the Divine Feminine energy to birth our baby in the world.

· I promise to let you hold me, support me, and love me with a heart of gratitude.

· I promise to walk the Gates of Transformation with courage and strength as I transition into Mother.

· I promise to honor my body and our baby's wishes, even if they are different from my own preferences.

_____
Signature and Date

I, Murray Moran, enter into Sacred Partnership with wife Alexandria Moran for the purpose of, together, birthing a baby into the world in the winter of 2019/2020 with love, trust, peace, and safety. For the duration of this pregnancy, throughout labor, delivery, and into the first three months of postpartum, I enter into these vows:

· I promise to be the dominant Divine Masculine energy of the birthing space for you to feel safe, held, protected, and at peace to labor as you need.

· I promise to remind you of how beautiful and powerful you are as a woman bringing our child into the world.

· I promise to keep a sense of groundedness and safety, even if things become chaotic.

· I promise to trust your instincts as a woman and a mother

· I promise to walk my own Gates of Transformation with courage and strength as I transition into Father.

_____
Signature and Date

Appendix III

Doula Tips to Have an Empowered Non-Medicated Birth

Over the past few years, there has been a rise in curiosity for non-medicated births and a slow movement toward a more traditional birthing experience. With this, comes a resurgence of traditional birthing techniques. There are many different coping mechanisms you can use to work through a non-medicated birth that will ease the pain, focus your mind, and help move labor along. Preparing for an empowered non-medicated birth by learning different methods and schools of thought will provide you with a well-rounded arsenal of tools to help walk you through the Gates of Transformation. One of the most important tools is understanding why you want to walk through the gates without any pain relief. Throughout this book, there are different practices and journal prompts that can help you uncover your emotional needs for your birth.

Here are our top doula tips to have the most empowering experience:

1. Understand Why You Want to Have a Non-Medicated Birth

This might seem like an odd step, but it's actually the most important. Understanding why you want to have a non-medicated birth allows you to emotionally connect to your preparation and to the experience itself. The Gates of Transformation take us on a journey of self-discovery, and the best way to start off that journey is to understand why you decided to take a certain path.

2. Work With a Doctor or Midwife Who Supports Your Choice

Finding a supportive medical team will allow for an environment that will embrace your views and cultivate an experience that feels safe. Surrounding yourself with professionals that respect you and your decisions will empower not only you, but also your Sacred Partner (see Chapter 6).

3. Preparation

This is one of the most important factors in having an empowered non-medicated birth. The collective cultural knowledge that was once ingrained in our minds has slowly faded. Learning about labor is key to walking through all the Gates of Transformation, so take a birthing class, watch positive birth videos, or hire a doula. Knowledge is power.

4. Consider a Doula or Someone with Birth Experience

One of the biggest challenges can be a lack of support. When you are walking through the Gates of Transformation, the guidance of a trustworthy partner creates a space of safety. Having someone to lean on when you are in labor shouldn't be a luxury; you deserve to be surrounded by those whom you love, honor, and support your choices. Better yet, create a Sacred Partnership (see Chapter 6) with someone who can help you achieve your full Goddess energy for an empowering experience.

5. Labor at Home as Long as Possible or Birth at Home

When trying to achieve an empowered and successful non-medicated birth, you must allow your mind, body, and soul to feel comfortable for as long as possible. The best way to do that is to stay at home for as long as possible, or better yet, birth at home.

If you are birthing in the hospital, staying at home as long as possible can mean something different for everyone, depending on who you are and how your labor is progressing. Traditionally, the rule is not to go to the hospital or birthing center until your contractions are five minutes apart, one minute in length for one full hour. By the time most women get to this part of their labor, they can transfer to the hospital without stalling labor and can keep progressing at a stable rate. Get to the hospital too soon and you are more likely to experience interventions with medications.

Appendix IV

Doula Tips to Have an
Empowered Epidural Birth

One of the best aspects of modern medicine is the ability to have an epidural during labor. An epidural can allow for the space to experience a gentle, and calm labor and delivery. However, even if you have an epidural, you'll still need to walk through The Gates of Transformation because it won't take away the emotional hurdles—these still have to be worked through.

Understanding why you want to have an epidural can be a key factor in how you walk through the Gates of Transformation. Throughout this book, there are exercises and journal prompts that will help guide your decision. This kind of self-work will create an empowered and informed mindset. By setting yourself up for emotional success, you will be able to communicate how you feel throughout your labor even if you aren't feeling your labor.

Here are our top doula tips to have the most empowering experience:

1. Understand Why You Want an Epidural

Understanding why you want to have an epidural allows you to emotionally connect to your preparation and to the experience itself. The Gates of Transformation takes us on a journey of self-discovery, and the best way to start off that journey is to understand why you decided to take a certain path. Be sure that your reasons are to help you walk through the gates rather than avoid them.

2. Preparation

Taking a birth class can really help you understand what an epidural is and how it affects your body, labor and baby. Talking to other mothers or doulas about their experiences can help you understand the process and how to achieve an empowered epidural experience.

3. Consider a Doula

Many people think you don't need a doula or an experienced birth worker if you're planning to have an epidural, but that isn't the case. When you receive an epidural, you still walk through all of the Gates of Transformation and need emotional support. Also, a doula can help suggest body positions and keep you moving to help progress your labor even if you are bedridden.

4. Focus on Your Energetic Birth Plan

When preparing for your birth, make sure you add that you want to have an empowered epidural. Go over with your Sacred Partner (see Chapter 6) what that means to you and how it can be accomplished. When you go into labor, focus your intentions on your Energetic Birth Plan.

5. Find a Doctor or Midwife Who Supports Your Choice

It's okay to interview more than one doctor or midwife. Many people think they should just stay with their first choice, but if your medical professional doesn't respect your choices, then they are not the right person for your birth. We understand you might not have a wide range of options, but finding someone who will listen to your wants and needs is important to have an empowered birth. If for some reason you are stuck with a medical professional that doesn't support your vision, you can use the energy of the Sacred Partner (see Chapter 6) to make the environment as supportive and empowering as possible.

Appendix V

Doula Tips to Have an Empowered Planned C-Section

The majority of planned C-sections are due to medical conditions or known risks identified in pregnancy; it can then be decided between the family and the medical team. In other circumstances, a planned C-section can be a result of a mother's or doctor's preference. In either circumstance, a planned C-section means mom schedules the baby's birth date and time with the surgeon a few weeks before her estimated due date to ensure that mom will not go into labor.

To have an empowered belly birth, you will want to make sure you still choose to walk through your Gates of Transformation from Maiden-to-Mother. With a planned C-section, you won't actually go into labor, so your gates will show up in pregnancy and in recovery. Just because you aren't laboring through your birth doesn't mean you get to bypass the sacrifices asked of this kind of transformation. You may even experience them more intensely than a tranditional vaginal birth or you may face each of the gates from the Gate of Courage and Sovereignty to the Gate of Intentional Surrender over and over again.

We highly recommend returning to the various chapters in this book as the gates show up in pregnancy to support yourself through your own belly birth labor process.

Here are our top doula tips to have the most empowering experience:

1. Understand the Medical Condition or Reason for Choosing a C-Section

Allowing your mind to understand what is happening on a physical level for you and your baby, as well as comprehending the risks, can help you find logical and mental acceptance—especially if this isn't your first-choice experience. If it is your first-choice experience, understanding your personal reasoning can help bring a fuller sense of validation.

2. Do Introspection Work to Uncover Any Hidden or Contradictory Emotions

Many moms facing a planned C-section find themselves battling conflicting and unexpected emotions. Feelings of confusion, anger, shame, and fear co-exist with feelings of hope, gratitude, joy, and relief, and this is all normal. Taking time to acknowledge and honor all your feelings can bring a deeper sense of acceptance and surrender before surgery occurs, so you are more likely to feel empowered as it is happening and focus on the blessing of having a baby.

3. Focus on Your Energetic Birth Plan

Just because a C-section is happening doesn't mean you have to abandon your Energetic Birth Plan. You can let your birth team and partner know that you still want to uphold the energy and intention of your Energetic Birth Plan (see Chapter 4) throughout surgery and recovery.

4. Learn Your Options

Just because you are having surgery doesn't mean you lose all options in your birth. Talk to your birth team about what options are available to help make your surgery feel like the birth you want. Research gentle cesarean methods to give you more information. Ask questions like:

- Can my birth partner or I have skin-to-skin as soon as the baby is born?
- Can I have just a spinal block or epidural rather than full anesthetic?
- How soon can I breastfeed—in the operating room or in recovery?
- Can I have delayed cord clamping?
- Can I have music in the operating room?
- Can someone take photos or video?

5. Learn About the C-Section Process and Surgery

Take a C-section class or research what happens in the surgery before you go in. This can be very helpful in feeling included in the surgery. Ask your doctor to tell you what they are doing as they do it. You don't have to be on the sidelines of this experience if you don't want to. Knowledge can often bring a greater sense of empowerment.

6. Walk Through Your Gates

The Gates of Transformation show up in different ways through this birth journey than they do in vaginal labor. Learn to recognize them along the way as often as you can. The more you can release your emotions and surrender while still having sovereignty, the more empowered you will feel during this beautiful birth experience.

Appendix VI

Doula Tips to Have an Empowered Emergency C-Section

The majority of emergency C-sections are just that—emergencies. As such, they often surprise us. Emergencies can bring on a lot of feelings that work against the experience of empowered birthing. Fear, shock, surprise, stress, disappointment, exhaustion, and shame are just a few of the common feelings a woman can feel when she is rushed into an emergency C-section. Very often, it can be a life-or-death situation, so the level of adrenaline and anxiety is high. So, the question is, how do you keep your sense of sovereignty and walk through the Gates of Transformation when something very scary is happening?

Our answer: preparation. In all of our prenatal appointments with our doula clients, especially those who are planning on a vaginal birth, we like to walk them through what an emergency C-section looks like. We do this for two reasons. First, by understanding what happens in a C-section, a lot of fear can dissipate, and this has a calming effect. When we know what to expect, the unexpected can seem less scary and more manageable. Second, by neutralizing any fears around cesarean births and showing how this kind of birth is also beautiful, moms find themselves more relaxed about their labors and able to surrender to how the birth unfolds. We hope that in reading the following doula tips, you too will be able to find empowerment in an emergency C-section scenario so should that happen to be your birth path, you are prepared.

We also believe that if a mom is walking through her Gates of Transformation in pregnancy and is getting acquainted with each sacrifice and surrender, she is also less likely to need one. But should you need one, you'll be prepared and practiced in the gates that show up, including the Gate of Expectations and the Gate of Intentional Surrender.

Here are our top doula tips to have the most empowering experience:

1. Learn About the C-Section Process in Pregnancy

Even if you plan to have a natural home or hospital birth, we highly recommend that you educate yourself on the C-section surgery and process. Take a C-section class or ask your doula or doctor to describe what happens in an emergency C-section. Make sure you are getting your information from a neutral source rather than from a friend who had a traumatizing experience. Knowing what the surgery is all about will help you feel less fearful of it and more empowered should it happen to you.

2. Focus on Your Energetic Birth Plan

Just because a C-section is happening, and even if your heart was set on a completely different kind of birth, that doesn't mean you have to abandon your Energetic Birth Plan (see Chapter 4). On the contrary, in an emergency situation, this is the one thing you can and should hold on to. As moms and Sacred Partners (see Chapter 6), you can focus on your intention for a loving birth experience, even if you are being rushed into the OR. This means finding courage, positivity, surrender, and acceptance very quickly. If you've been practicing walking through the Gates of Transformation in pregnancy, it should be a little easier to dobso in an emergency situation.

3. Rely on Your Sacred Partner

An emergency C-section is where your Sacred Partner can really shine and where you can really walk through the Gate of Sacred Partnership (see Chapter 6). This is where that supportive, encouraging, and validating Divine Masculine energy can help ground you and focus your attention on the positivity. Ask your Sacred Partner to peek over the sheet and tell you what is happening to help you feel included. Have your Sacred Partner talk about the baby. Say things like, "I wonder what his/her/their little fingers will look like . . . what color hair do you think the baby will have?" This may help keep your mind off the "emergency" and more on the birth. This requires great strength and preparation on behalf of the Sacred Partner to be this grounding force amidst the chaos of an emergency.

4. Focus on Bonding

As soon as you can, and are allowed to by your medical team, we recommend holding your baby and beginning the breastfeeding journey, if that's your choice. Be present, talk to your baby, and continue to emit the energy of your Energetic Birth Plan. If your baby has to be in the NICU, then have your Sacred Partner go with the baby and be there, holding that intention. As soon as you and baby can be together, focus on bonding, and connection.

5. Process the Birth Experience When You Can

With all emergency experiences, it is really important to process the experience mentally, emotionally, and spiritually. You can talk through what happened with your doctor, doula, partner, friend, pediatrician, or therapist. Tell your birth story, your feelings, your experience. Write it, draw it, sing it. Allow your body to move through any possible trauma or stuckness so you can feel more empowered as you move into motherhood.

Recommended Resources

Childbirth and Labor

Birth Works International, https://www.birthworks.org
International Cesarean Awareness Network, https://www.ican-online.org
Evidence-Based Birth, https://evidencebasedbirth.com
Waterbirth International, https://www.waterbirth.org

Childbirth Education

Birthing from Within, https://www.birthingfromwithin.com
Hypnobirthing—the Morgan Method, https://www.hypnobirthing.com
The Bradley Method, http://bradleybirth.com/

Positive Birth Books and Stories

Birth Without Fear: The Judgment-Free Guide to Taking Charge of Your Pregnancy, Birth, and Postpartum by January Harshe (Hachette, 2019)
Sacred Birthing: Birthing a New Humanity, 2nd ed., by Sunni Karll, D.D. (CreateSpace, 2017)
Ina May's Guide to Childbirth by Ina May Gaskin (Bantam-Random House, 2003)
Orgasmic Birth: Your Guide to a Safe, Satisfying, and Pleasurable Birth Experience by Elizabeth Davis and Debra Pascali-Bonaro (Rodale, 2010)

Finding a Doula

DONA International, https://www.dona.org
CAPPA, https://www.cappa.net
National Black Doulas Association, https://blackdoulas.org

Birth Trauma

Sage Therapeutics, https://www.postpartumdepression.com
The Birth Trauma Association, https://www.birthtraumaassociation.org.uk
Postpartum Support International, https://www.postpartum.net

Energetic or Womb Healing

National Board for Certified Clinical Hypnotherapists, http://www.natboard.com
From Womb to World, http://www.fromwombtoworld.com
The Spirit Baby Collective, http://www.soulbabycommunication.com

References

1   Czarnocka J, Slade P. "Prevalence and predictors of post-traumatic stress symptoms following childbirth." *Br J Clin Psychol*, 2000. 39 (Pt 1):35–51.

2   American Friends of Tel Aviv University. "One in three post-partum women suffers PTSD symptoms after giving birth: Natural births a major cause of post-traumatic stress, study suggests." *ScienceDaily*. www.sciencedaily.com/releases/2012/08/120808121949.htm (accessed September 2, 2019).

3   ETH Zurich. "Hereditary trauma: Inheritance of traumas and how they may be mediated." *ScienceDaily*. www.sciencedaily.com/releases/2014/04/140413135953.htm (accessed September 3, 2019).

4   Lumley MA, Cohen JL, Borszcz GS, Cano A, Radcliffe AM, Porter LS, Schubiner H, Keefe FJ. "Pain and emotion: a biopsychosocial review of recent research." *J Clin Psychol*. 2011 Sep. 67(9):942–68. doi: 10.1002/jclp.20816. Epub 2011 Jun 6. PMID: 21647882; PMCID: PMC3152687.

5   Dunkel Schetter C, Tanner L. "Anxiety, depression and stress in pregnancy: implications for mothers, children, research, and practice." *Curr Opin Psychiatry*. 2012 Mar. 25(2):141–8. doi: 10.1097/YCO.0b013e3283503680. PMID: 22262028; PMCID: PMC4447112. https://www.ncbi.nlm.nih.gov/pmc/articles/PMC4447112/

6   Tierney AL, Nelson CA 3rd. "Brain Development and the Role of Experience in the Early Years. Zero Three." 2009 Nov. 1;30(2):9-13. PMID: 23894221; PMCID: PMC3722610. https://doi.org/10.1177/0956797611422073. Volume: 23 issue: 1, page(s): 93–100

7   Werner, E. A., Myers, M. M., Fifer, W. P., Cheng, B., Fang, Y., Allen, R. and Monk, C. (2007), Prenatal predictors of infant temperament. Dev. Psychobiol., 49: 474-484. doi:10.1002/dev.20232

8   Pearlstein, T., Howard, M., Salisbury, A., & Zlotnick, C. "Postpartum depression." *American Journal of Obstetrics and Gynecology*. 2009. 200(4), 357–364. doi:10.1016/j.ajog.2008.11.033 https://www.ncbi.nlm.nih.gov/pmc/articles/PMC3918890/

9   Onoye, J. M., Shafer, L. A., Goebert, D. A., Morland, L. A., Matsu, C. R., & Hamagami, F. "Changes in PTSD symptomatology and mental health during pregnancy and postpartum." Archives of women's mental health. 2013. 16(6): 453–463. doi:10.1007/s00737-013-0365-8. https://www.ncbi.nlm.nih.gov/pmc/articles/PMC3888817/

Bibliography

Afua Q. *Sacred Woman: A Guide to Healing the Feminine Body, Mind, and Spirit*. New York, NY: One World Books; 2000.

Chapman G. *The 5 Love Languages: The Secrets to Love That Lasts*. Rev ed. Chicago, IL: Northfield Publishing; 2015.

Daulter A. *Sacred Pregnancy: A Loving Guide and Journal for Expectant Moms*. Berkeley, CA: North Atlantic Books; 2012.

Davis E, Pascali-Bonaro D. *Orgasmic Birth: Your Guide to a Safe, Satisfying, and Pleasurable Birth Experience*. New York, NY: Rodale Inc; 2010.

England P. *Ancient Map for Modern Birth: Preparation, Passage, and Personal Growth for the Childbearing Year*. Albuquerque, NM: Seven Gates Media; 2017.

England P, Horowitz R. *Birthing From Within: An Extra-Ordinary Guide to Childbirth Preparation*. Albuquerque, NM: Partera Press; 1998.

Gaskin IM. *Ina May's Guide to Childbirth*. New York, NY: Bantam Books; 2003.

Harshe J. *Birth Without Fear: The Judgement-Free Guide to Taking Charge of Your Pregnancy, Birth, and Postpartum*. New York, NY: Hachette Books; 2019.

Johnson KA. *The Fourth Trimester: A Postpartum Guide to Healing Your Body, Balancing Your Emotions and Restoring Your Vitality*. Boulder, CO: Shambhala Publications; 2017.

Karll S. *Sacred Birthing: Birthing a New Humanity*. 2nd ed. CreateSpace; 2017.

Kleiman KR, Raskin VD. *This Isn't What I Expected: Overcoming Postpartum Depression.* 2nd ed. Boston, MA: Da Capo Press; 2013.

Marquis M, Francis EA. *Witchy Mama: Magickal Traditions, Motherly Insights and Sacred Knowledge.* Woodbury, MN: Llewellyn Publications; 2016.

Verny TR, Weintraub P. *Pre-Parenting: Nurturing Your Child From Conception.* New York, NY: Simon & Schuster; 2002.

Acknowledgments

There are a few people who have been on this journey with us as we traveled into the Underworld of authorship to birth the wisdom within these pages and transform ourselves from birth doulas to messengers. Without these brave and supportive souls, walking alongside us through the Gates of Transformation, this book would never have been birthed into existence. For your support, love, and encouragement, we are forever thankful.

First and foremost, let us thank the amazing, brave, and powerful women who have honored us with their vulnerability and trust in birth. Your courage, sacrifice, struggles, and victories have each made a significant impact on the wisdom shared in this book. Thank you for allowing us to tell your stories, teaching us the great truths of the feminine, and being the trailblazers for this new way of seeing birth. You are all goddesses!

To our families who have been the rock-solid ground, we found ourselves needing throughout the book writing process. A few individuals deserve special thanks:

To Douglas Mahana, thank you for allowing me to finally find my true passion. You have been a pillar of strength and love throughout this experience. Thank you for being my partner in life and father to our daughters. You have shown me what the Divine Masculine can be. I love you.

To Rosalind Mahana thank you for making me a mother. It's true what they say . . . you don't know what love is until you have a child. And you gave me that. Thank you for being patient with Mommy while I spent our "quiet time" writing. You allowed me the space to be creative, and I love you for that.

To Lilian Mahana, this book would not be here without you, your little spirit helped wield this divine work into being. Being pregnant while writing this book was an amazing experience, and you helped guide me through the Gates of Transformation with strength and grace. I love you.

To the women in my family, Mom, Emily, and Enna thank you for the love and support you have given me throughout the years. I wouldn't be the woman I am today without you.

A big thank you to Murray Moran for the late nights of proofreading, the constant encouragement, the endless wiping away of tears of frustration, and especially showing me and the world what it means to be a man, embodied in his divine self. This book would never have made it off the pages of the heart onto the pages here without your fierce belief in us and in the power of the Divine Feminine. I can't do life without you.

To Oliver Moran, for teaching me the powerful lessons of surrender, trust, and acceptance not only in birth but also in motherhood. I feel so blessed to be your mommy.

To Gina Fuschetto, our creative goddess, who helped bring to life the image, art, and brand of this book. Your countless hours of love and talent have blessed us beyond words. You have truly animated the essence of the message.

To Chrystal Rhea, who opened doors we didn't know were there and introduced us to an amazing editor. Thank you for being a great friend and female supporter.

To Sandy Draper for reshaping our words and editing our book in a way that brings greater love, clarity, acceptance, and inclusivity to the energy of the book. Your talent and work are deeply cherished.

And finally, to Hay House and Balboa Press for giving our book a chance to be shared with the world.

Lauren Mahana and Alexandria Moran

About the Author

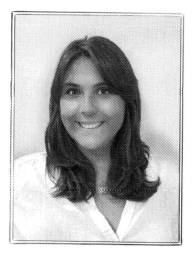

Lauren Mahana

Lauren Mahana is a practicing birth doula, intuitive healer, wife, and mother of two daughters living in New York City. When Lauren was 16 years old, she was gifted her first tarot deck; it was the start of a long, winding journey down a spiritual path. Through most of her late teens and 20s, Lauren was lost living in NYC; she started and ended many different paths, from multiple colleges, retail jobs, the restaurant world, and merchandising, and she began to wonder why nothing seemed to stick. Lauren then decided to find work that would feed her soul, first and foremost.

She began working at a local Brooklyn herb shop, which ignited her spiritual path. While studying herbalism, Reiki, shamanic healing, flower essences, and essential oils, Lauren realized that her path was known all along—she was a healer. She first focused on a small herbal practice and then integrated her practice with Reiki and tarot. After becoming a mother, she found a calling to help guide other women during birth. Becoming a birth doula was the perfect cap on the direction of what has officially become her Intuitive Healing Practice.

For the past 10 years, Lauren has been exploring, studying, and practicing to be a well-rounded healer. Her passion comes from her drive to help heal the wounds of the spirit so the collective can be transformed.

About the Author

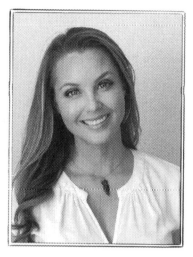

Alexandria Moran

Alexandria Moran is a practicing spiritual healer, women's empowerment coach, and trained clairvoyant psychic. She is the creator of Witch + Womb, an online community for women to gather, heal, and witness each other through all aspects and phases of womanhood (including conception, pregnancy, childbirth, and postpartum). Her business focuses on helping women heal their spiritual and emotional traumas around femininity and womanhood.

Through her work, she has discovered that a woman's birth experience stays with her forever and shapes the woman on a deep core level. Her experience as a birth doula, postpartum doula, childbirth educator, birth photographer, and mother has allowed Alexandria to understand labor and birth as so much more than *just* a medical or physical experience. It is truly the greatest spiritual opportunity for women to heal themselves and their own lineage. She's found that birth—when labored in empowerment, courage, and intentional surrender—is truly an initiation into a higher level of consciousness for humanity.

Through her work with pregnant and postpartum women, she's become passionate about helping women avoid birth trauma, PTSD, and postpartum depression before it happens.

Her main goal is to help women navigate their own subconscious and spiritual blocks during pregnancy, so they are prepared on all levels of the labor experience. The tools put forth in this book are a culmination of her life's work around trauma healing, spiritual acknowledgment, and honoring of the Divine Feminine.

Index

Notes

Notes

Notes

Notes